# Juicing for Health

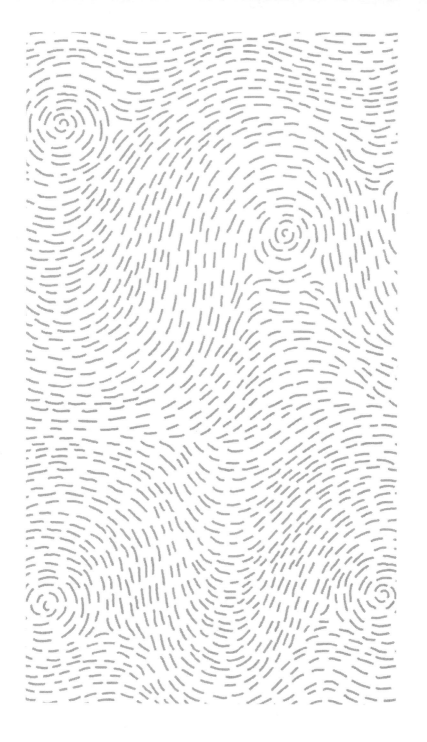

# JUICING
## *for Health*

**81** JUICING RECIPES

AND **76** INGREDIENTS

PROVEN TO IMPROVE

HEALTH AND VITALITY

MENDOCINO
PRESS

For general information on our other products and services or to obtain technical support, please contact our Customer Care Department within the United States at (866) 744-2665, or outside the United States at (510) 253-0500.

Mendocino Press publishes its books in a variety of electronic and print formats. Some content that appears in print may not be available in electronic books, and vice versa.

ISBN: Print 978-1-62315-330-4 | eBook 978-1-62315-331-1

## Chapter Four: Juicing Cleanse and Detox Plans    67

Three-Day Pure Juice Cleanse Plan    69

Seven-Day Detox Challenge    71

**PART TWO**

# Recipes for Health

## Chapter Five: General Health and Well-Being    77

Achy Breaky Muscles    78

Balancing Act    80

Beet Cramps    82

Beet the Heat    84

Bladder Infection Be Gone    86

Carrot Colon Cleanse    88

Clean as a Whistle Kidney Cleanse    90

Clean Artery Sweep    92

Garden Fresh Blast    94

Great Grapefruit Cleanse    96

Green Joint Relief    98

Heart Beet    100

LDL Reducer    102

Healthy Prostate Blend    104

Love Boost    106

Spinach Sugar Stabilizer    108

Stimulating Sunshine    110

Healthy Heart Summer Salad    112

Under Pressure    114

## Chapter Six: Immune System Support    117

Citrus Cough Buster    118

Superfood Detox    120

Flu Fighter    122

Full System Boost    124

# Contents

Introduction   1

**PART ONE**

## Juicing for Health

### Chapter One: Juicing Basics   5
What Is Juicing?   5
Health Benefits of Juicing   7
Buying a Juicer   9
Technique Tips   12
FAQ about Juicing   13

### Chapter Two: Nature's Pharmacy   19
Fruit Juice versus Vegetable Juice   20
Healing Fruits   21
Healing Vegetables   33
The Toxic Twenty   45
Healing Add-Ins   48
Potent Combinations   54
Seven Tips for Making Great Juices   54

### Chapter Three: Juice Cleansing for Health   57
What Is a Juice Cleanse?   57
Benefits of a Cleanse   59
Is a Cleanse Right for You?   61
Tips for a Safe and Successful Cleanse   62

Getting a Boost        126
Kick the Cold        128
Sage Advice for Sore Throat        130
Splendid Sinuses        132

## Chapter Seven: Weight Loss and Digestion Enhancers        135
Acid Away        136
Bye-Bye Nausea        138
Does a Body Good        140
Easy Digestion        142
Get Things Moving        144
Good Morning        146
Green Heartburn Relief        148
Gut Flora Builder        150
IBS Support        152
Meal in a Glass        154
Metabolism Mover        156
Papaya Gut Reprieve        158

## Chapter Eight: Cancer and Disease Prevention        161
Better Body        162
Bonny Bone Fruit Surprise        164
Cutting Cancer        166
Gout Be Gone        168
Happy Colon        170
Healthful Heart Ginger        172
Promote Prostate Health        174
Beat Breast Cancer        176
Thyroid Buddy        178

## Chapter Nine: Energy and Vitality Boost        181
Aftermath Recovery        182
Before Gym Blitz        184
Burn, Baby, Burn        186

Fat Furnace     188

Green Go-Go     190

Pick Me Up     192

Ready to Recover     194

Slow Energy     196

## Chapter Ten: Taming Inflammation     199

Allergy Relief     200

Asparagus Arthritis Relief     202

Breathe Easy     204

Glowing Ginseng     206

Inflammation Buster     208

Liquid Chlorophyll     210

Minty Fennel     212

Passionately Immune     214

Perky Parsnip     216

Simply Wheatgrass     218

Vital MS Support     220

## Chapter Eleven: Mind, Brain, and Mental Wellness     223

Apple Alzheimer's Prevention     224

Clearly Cabbage     226

Focus on Hydration     228

Happy in a Glass     230

Healthful Headache Remedy     232

Rosy Relaxer     234

Sweet Dreams     236

## Chapter Twelve: Beauty and Skin Enhancers     239

Beeting Eczema     240

Carrot Clear-Up     242

Circle Banisher     244

Citrus Cellulite Be Gone    246

Lots of Locks    248

Shiny Tresses    250

Vanishing Veins    252

**References**    255

**Index**    259

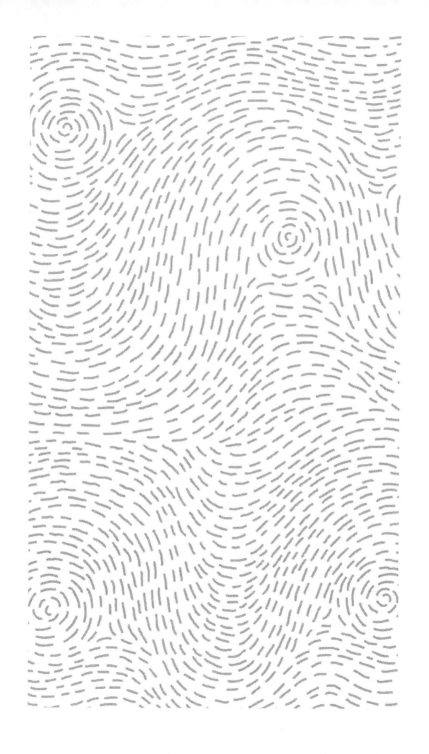

# Introduction

I f you have ever had orange juice squeezed from sun-warmed fruit right off the tree, you will understand why so many people are juicing every carrot, apple, and tomato in their kitchen. The juice simply tastes better, like holding sunshine and lazy summer days right in your hand. It should be no surprise that fresh juice is also much more nutritious than commercially processed products. Juicing has become a popular way to get the goodness and health-boosting components of fruit and vegetables.

Learning to juice is not difficult. But it may be expensive and confusing if you jump right in without knowing what's the best juicer for your needs or what combination of fruits and vegetables will address your acne or insomnia. Without a little direction and advice, you might find yourself creating some truly unpalatable juices that will turn you away from juicing forever! This book is organized so that you first learn the basics of juicing, the health benefits you can expect when juicing, and the answers to some common questions, before delving into the building blocks of your juices—a vast array of delicious fruits, vegetables, herbs, and spices—and the unique healing characteristics of each ingredient.

In this book you will find all the information you need to start juicing for health, ranging from what type of juicer might be right for you all the way to the specific nutrients in each berry or carrot. Once you understand the power of juicing and the impact wonderful fresh juices can have on your body, it is time to discover juice cleanses and detoxing so you can eliminate dangerous toxins. Vital information about who should not go on a juice cleanse, the health benefits of detoxing, and valuable strategies for successful cleanses are all here for easy reference.

To make your first cleanse effective and positive, use the easy-to-follow three-day juice cleanses and seven-day detox challenge meal plans found in this book. These plans use the recipes found in Part Two, and are designed for a system-wide detox. If you want to address a particular organ or health problem with your cleanse, mix and match the recipes to create a tailored plan. The recipes are divided into categories targeting specific health concerns, and each recipe is followed by a list of additional fruits and vegetables you may use to make your own targeted juice blends.

Food is a very powerful weapon against disease. Including juicing as part of your regular routine puts you on the path to vibrant good health.

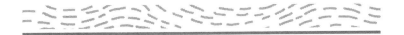

PART ONE

# Juicing for Health

CHAPTER ONE: JUICING BASICS

CHAPTER TWO: NATURE'S PHARMACY

CHAPTER THREE: JUICE CLEANSING FOR HEALTH

CHAPTER FOUR: JUICING CLEANSE AND DETOX PLANS

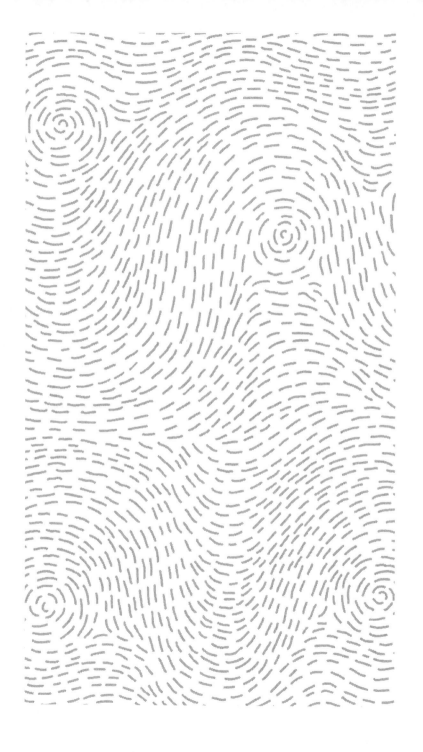

# Juicing Basics

Juicing is not a new phenomenon that became popular because of advances in science, or because someone lost weight juicing and they wanted to tell the world. Juicing is actually centuries old, and is even mentioned in the Dead Sea Scrolls as a way to get "profound strength and subtle form" from figs and pomegranates. South Asian cultures have used juicing for centuries to make healing beverages as a part of the medical system known as Ayurveda. Juicing is not a fad or a trend; it is an accepted practice used to get valuable nutrients into the body efficiently.

The equipment for juicing has certainly changed with respect to separating pulp from juice. Modern scientific studies have also pinpointed very specific benefits provided by juicing, as this book will discuss. Since juicing is so mainstream now, it has never been easier to incorporate juicing into your life and start reaping the benefits.

## WHAT IS JUICING?

Juicing means extracting the juice from fruits, vegetables, and herbs, using a juicer machine. All your produce and herbs go into the juicer raw, and you will even be juicing stems, skins, and seeds in some cases. This practice has become very popular in the past few years, as these fresh concentrated juices have been linked to countless health benefits. But why juice at all when you can get commercially produced juice in every combination in the local supermarket? The main reason to juice is simply that prepared juices cannot match the level of quality of fresh juice, not to mention the fact that store-bought juices are usually pasteurized, which destroys many nutrients, enzymes, and minerals. Plus, there is nothing quite as tasty as a glass of juice just extracted from a ripe peach or carrot.

When you begin juicing in your own home, rather than simply picking up a carton of juice at the store, you may be surprised to find that it takes a very large quantity of produce to make a single serving of juice. You will be processing and juicing a few pounds of fresh fruits and vegetables to make about sixteen ounces of juice, and there will be cleanup involved. Is all this fuss worth it?

The cornerstone of vibrant good health is getting enough vegetables and fruits into your diet every single day—about nine servings—and most people fall short of that goal. Juicing is a wonderful way to incorporate all those servings into your meals and reap the rewards of all the accessible nutrients.

Unless you are doing a juice cleanse, these extracted juices should not replace fresh whole fruits and vegetables—you should be eating these as well. Juicing extracts the juice from the produce but leaves behind the fiber, which plays a very important role in digestion, blood sugar regulation, and the cardiovascular system. You want to make sure to get enough fiber as well as nutrients, so make sure your diet is balanced between juices and solid foods. You will be juicing your produce and herbs raw, sometimes with the stems, skin, and seeds included. Using every part offers health benefits you might not get when cooking, peeling, and coring your produce. For example, many nutrients are found right under the skin or in the skin on some fruits and vegetables, such as cucumbers, and in the seeds of other produce, such as protein in cantaloupe.

There are countless health benefits associated with juicing, from a reduced risk of chronic diseases such as cancer and diabetes to clearer skin and shiny hair. If you want to get healthier and perhaps try to help manage an existing health condition, juicing might be the solution for you.

## HEALTH BENEFITS OF JUICING

Juicing can take many forms, from adding a couple of fresh juices a day or every few days to your diet, all the way to consuming only fresh juices for days at a time. How much you want to juice is up to you and your doctor. There are health benefits associated with all ranges of juicing, even at the minimum end of the range. This is because fruits and vegetables are the foundation of good health, and juicing allows even the most committed carnivore the opportunity to get the daily recommended amount of fruits and vegetables. If you decide to start juicing only once a day, you can still expect to reap many benefits.

- The entire point of juicing is to give your digestive tract and associated organs involved in digestion, energy production, and waste control (colon, kidneys, liver, bladder, intestines) a break. This leads to a healthier digestive system.
- Juicing removes the fiber from your fruits and vegetables, which allows instant absorption of nutrients and a quick conversion to energy in the blood. The energy spent on digestion and converting food to blood sugar, about 30 percent in the body, can be diverted to other activities. This means you will have more energy and stamina on the days you have fresh juice.
- The quick absorption of nutrients means they are delivered more quickly to cells, facilitating any repair and healing.
- Easily accessible antioxidants from many different fruits and vegetables can quickly reduce the damage caused by free radicals in the blood, as well as reduce the risk of cancer, heart disease, diabetes, asthma, and autoimmune diseases.
- Regular juicing with a range of vibrant, colorful produce, which contain many nutrients as well as antioxidants, can reduce the risk of age-related diseases, such as macular degeneration, cataracts, and arthritis.

- Thanks to many immunity boosting vitamins and nutrients found in juices, you'll have a stronger immune system that is able to fight off more serious health problems as well as the common cold and flu.
- Expect an improved memory and better cognitive function well into your older years, due to the antioxidant action of fruits and vegetables, which minimizes free radical damage to cells in the brain.
- Enjoy a more robust sex drive, because the nutrients in juices help balance hormones and improve blood flow, which in turn increases libido.

**If you have ever had a cut become inflamed and red, you have seen a process called oxidation in practice.** Oxidation is a natural process that happens when oxygen reacts to cells, and it causes changes to occur like fresh new skin to replace the damaged skin. However, about 2 percent of the time this change creates damaged cells, which are called free radicals. These cells are missing a molecule, which makes them "steal" molecules from healthy cells, damaging the DNA of the healthy cell and creating mutated cells. These mutant cells multiply abnormally, supplying an opening for diseases like cancer. The thousands of antioxidants (nutrients and enzymes) in fruits and vegetables are crucial for defending the body against free radicals by stopping this damaging chain reaction either before or after it starts. An assortment of different antioxidants are needed to fully protect the body, because each works in a different way. Vitamin E breaks a chain reaction that has already begun and vitamin C stops it before it starts. Antioxidants need to be constantly replenished, because when they neutralize free radicals, they become oxidized themselves.

## BUYING A JUICER

So you are excited about incorporating fresh extracted juices into your diet, and maybe even want to try a juice cleanse. You first need to figure out what kind of juicer to buy. This is not a small decision, because juicers can be expensive and you don't want to buy the SUV of juicers when what you really need is a compact.

There are some questions you need to consider before making your purchase. To pinpoint your juicing needs, here are some questions to consider.

- How much juicing will you actually be doing, daily or weekly?
- How much juice do you want to produce?
- What types of fruits and vegetables will you need to juice?
- What is your budget?
- How important is easy cleaning to you?
- Can you usually figure out complicated appliances or do you want something simple?
- Do you mind if your produce is heated up a little in the juicing process?
- Do you mind if a juicer is loud?
- How long do you want the juicer to last?

The answers to these questions will help you ascertain the right size, power, and price of your juicer. There are three basic types of juicers, and they are usually differentiated by the way they extract and separate the juice of your fruits and vegetables from the pulp.

### Centrifugal Juicers

These are generally the most inexpensive juicers. This type of juicer can juice any type of fruit or vegetable quickly but gets less of a juice yield out of leafy greens like spinach, wheatgrass, kale, and herbs. Each model of juicer is slightly different, and feeding chute size varies; some accept whole fruits and some are smaller, which means you have to cut up your produce to feed it into the juicer. Of the three main types of juicers, this type is the fastest and typically allows you to juice the biggest pieces of produce, sometimes whole fruits and vegetables.

In a centrifugal juicer, the fruit or vegetable is pushed through the chute, grated into a pulp, and then spun at a very high speed against a strainer screen, using centrifugal force to extract the juice. The juice comes out one side and the pulp is either left inside the machine for you to clean out, or comes out the opposite side.

Some things to consider about a centrifugal juicer include the fact that it is less efficient than other types of juicers, ejecting a wetter pulp, which means nutrients and juice are being cast out the waste side of the machine. Furthermore, the juice produced in a centrifugal juicer ends up with oxygen dissolved into it, because it is spun around at such high speeds. This added oxygen means the juice has a shorter shelf life and spoils quicker. You will need to drink your juice right away to avoid wasting it. These juicers are also quite loud, and the speed at which they rotate to extract the juice produces some heat inside the chamber. This means a small loss of nutrients due to a mild "cooking" process, which might bother you if you are a raw food purist. Some brands also generate foam, which means some of your nutrients are being lost in the froth.

· · · · · · · · · · · · · · · · · · · · · · · · · · · · · · · · · · · · · · · · · · · · · · · · ·

**It takes a great deal of produce to make one 8-ounce glass of juice, no matter what type of juicer you use. For example:**

1 cucumber = ¾ cup juice

1 head celery = 1¼ cups juice

2 big bunches spinach = ½ cup juice

8 medium carrots = 1 cup juice

1 large beet with greens = ½ cup juice

· · · · · · · · · · · · · · · · · · · · · · · · · · · · · · · · · · · · · · · · · · · · · · · · ·

## Masticating Juicers

These juicers, also called single gear or single auger, use an auger (a tool for boring holes) to chew up the produce in a grinding motion that breaks up more fiber than a centrifugal juicer. The juice is then extracted from the pulp by crushing the ground-up produce against a screen. The juice comes out one side and the pulp exits through a separate chute.

Masticating juicers extract more juice than centrifugal juicers do, as is evident by the much drier pulp. They can also easily process any type of vegetable, fruit, herb, leafy green, or grass. The quality of the juice from this type of juicer is very good.

Masticating juicers are not as fast as centrifugal juicers, so there is no heat produced or foam in the final product, and they are much quieter. The juice is less apt to spoil; it may be stored for up to forty-eight hours in the refrigerator in an airtight glass jar. Masticating juicers often serve double duty, because with attachments they can also make nut butters, baby foods, purées, and sauces as well as juices.

The downside of these versatile machines is that they are, on average, more expensive than centrifugal juicers, and it may take more time to make your juices. You will usually have to spend more time preparing your produce as well, because the feeding chute on masticating juicers is much smaller. That means feeding in chopped produce rather than whole.

## Triturating Juicers

This top-of-the-line juicer is similar to a masticating juicer, except instead of one gear or auger, there are two. The produce is ground up between two rolling augers, moving quite slowly, which means the juice is extracted efficiently and without heat, producing the greatest juice yield and nutrient quantity. This juicer produces the best juice possible. Similar to the masticating juicer, you can juice anything in the triturating juicer except perhaps pineapple, which does not go through efficiently because it is so very fibrous.

The triturating juicer is quiet and adds no foam or heat to the finished juice, therefore allowing for a longer refrigerator shelf life. With attachments, it may also produce purées, sauces, baby foods, and pâtés. The downside of this superior machine is that it is the most expensive of all the electric juicers. It also requires your fruits and vegetables to be cut into small pieces before they can be juiced, and it takes more time to juice.

In addition to centrifugal, masticating, and triturating juicers, there are smaller and specific juicers, such as wheatgrass juicers and hand juicers. The wheatgrass juicer is really only for wheatgrass, so you will not need one if you don't plan on juicing a great deal of wheatgrass, or if you have masticating or triturating juicers that can handle the grasses. Hand juicers are inexpensive and are great for juicing citrus fruit quickly, with no peeling or seed extraction. Hand juicers are perfect for occasional tasks, and cleanup is a snap, but they will not meet all your juicing needs.

## TECHNIQUE TIPS

No matter what type of juicer you decide to get to access the incredible health benefits of fresh, nutrient-rich juices in your own kitchen, the important part is to get something and start juicing. Here are some tips and techniques you can use, no matter what type of juicer you have.

- Always wash your hands and your produce thoroughly before juicing, because the finished products will not be pasteurized. This means bacteria are free to grow in your juice if you are not scrupulously clean and don't take precautions.
- Make sure your juicer is immaculately clean. Get into the habit of washing it immediately after juicing. This will prevent it from getting stained, and the task will be simpler without dried bits of fruit and vegetable in the chutes and body of the machine.

- If your juicer has a pulp bin for the discarded pulp, line it with a waste bag for easy cleanup.
- Prepare all your ingredients before you start to juice. The amount of prep will depend on the type of juicer you are using; masticating and triturating juicers require more chopping of fruit and vegetables to fit the feeding chutes.
- After you have finished juicing all your ingredients, let the juicer run a little longer to clean out the gears and centrifugal chamber and to allow the last drop of juice to come out.

## FAQ ABOUT JUICING

Perhaps you have heard a lot about juicing and might have even tried it. You might have some questions concerning the process, health benefits, side effects, and whether you should try a fast or just drink fresh juices as an addition to your diet. Here are some frequently asked questions about juicing.

**Isn't it healthier to just eat fruits and vegetables?**

It is very healthful to eat fresh produce, but sometimes the body needs to do a lot of work to access and use the nutrients found in fruits and vegetables. Digestion is hard work, and the fiber in fruit and vegetables can sweep nutrients out when it is excreted. With juicing, the nutrients are immediately accessible for the body to use.

**Will I lose weight when juicing?**

Some people lose weight when juicing. But some juices may have a lot of calories, so unless you are following a fast, you might exceed the amount of calories needed to support weight loss. If you are juice fasting to lose weight, it is important to consider that this type of diet is not sustainable long term, and any weight lost might come back when you end the fast.

**How long can I juice?**

You can juice indefinitely if you add fresh juices to a healthful diet as an accent or to target a specific health concern with a huge influx of nutrients. A juice fast should be done only after discussing it with your doctor, and only if it is done in a manner that is well planned, with all nutrient needs considered.

**Can I juice all parts of my fruits and vegetables?**

This is entirely up to you, but there are some skins, rinds, and seeds that should be removed for health or aesthetic reasons. The skin or rind and the flesh right under them may contain many nutrients, so they should be juiced whenever possible. Some ingredients you might want to peel are: kiwis, citrus fruits, papayas, avocados, butternut squashes, melons, and mangos. You should also take out the pits from mangos and stone fruits such as cherries, peaches, and papayas (because the stones are bitter). Always wash your fruit and vegetables thoroughly, even if they are organic, to remove any dirt, pesticides, or environmental contaminants.

**Did you know that apple seeds contain a substance that turns into hydrogen cyanide, a lethal poison, when metabolized?** Many people do not juice the cores of their apples for this reason. It would take more than one bushel of ground-up apple seeds to contain enough poison to kill an adult, though, so if you occasionally juice the whole apple, you should be fine.

**If I am detoxing, do I drink only fresh juices?**

The idea behind detoxing is to give your body a break from digesting food and to flush out toxins. Eating solid food during a detox will slow or stall that goal. You do not eat solid foods when detoxing.

**What amount of juice do I drink in a day if I am doing a cleanse?**

You need to alternate fresh juices and lots of water when fasting. Water is crucial for flushing toxins and helping cleanse the body. You should try to drink a combination of different juices in 16- to 20-ounce portions, four to six times a day.

**Do I have to drink the juice right away or can I store it?**

It is always best to drink your juices right away, because the nutrient value drops as it sits, and there is a chance of bacterial contamination. If you want to store your juice, use airtight glass jars and put the juice in the refrigerator for only about a day and in the freezer for no more than a week.

**Do I need to mix water into my juices?**

You don't need to dilute your juices at all, unless you find the flavor too strong.

**Do I need to take supplements when doing a juice cleanse?**

Supplements are used when you are not getting enough nutrients from your diet. But since juicing floods the body with many nutrients, you will simply overload your system with a supplement.

**Can I juice in a blender?**

Blending and juicing are different processes. Blending does not remove the fiber, which is part of the point of juicing. Blenders can be wonderful for smoothies, which may be consumed as an accompaniment to healthful juicing.

**If I'm juice cleansing, how do I get protein?**

There is lots of protein in dark, leafy greens and other produce, which can be accessed with juicing. For example, kale and romaine have about 7 grams of protein per serving, and spinach, asparagus, celery, and cauliflower have about 4 grams per serving.

**Is it normal for my urine and stool to be a weird color?**

This is a normal side effect of juicing. The color of your juices (green, red, purple, and orange) may often come out in what you excrete from your body.

**Can I juice if I have diabetes?**

Before considering juicing, you need to consult a doctor, especially if you are on medication for your condition. You should not fast or cleanse with juice when you are diabetic, but including vegetable-based juices once a day or several times a week could be beneficial.

**Can I take premade juices to work?**

It is best to drink your juices immediately, but you may take them with you if you have a refrigerator to store them in or a cooler to carry them safely.

**Do I need to buy organic produce exclusively?**

Organic fruits and vegetables are a good idea, especially if the ingredients fall in the toxic twenty (see the list in Chapter Two). Organic produce also tastes better and has more nutrients in some cases. Organic is not necessary, though, as long as you wash your ingredients thoroughly.

**Can I drink coffee or tea when doing a juice fast?**

You should avoid beverages that contain caffeine when detoxing, because caffeine is actually a toxin. You may drink any herbal teas.

**Can I exercise when doing a juice cleanse?**

You may exercise if you already have a regular workout plan, but keep in mind that muscles need protein to support activity and you may not be taking in enough for intense physical activity. Keep your exercise levels moderate to light when cleansing, and drink lots of water.

**What side effects can I expect when doing a juice cleanse?**

During the first few days you might experience physical discomfort associated with detoxing, especially if you were not a big consumer of fruit and vegetables to begin with before the cleanse. These side effects will fade away after a few days. You might experience:

• Body odor
• Constipation or diarrhea
• Dizziness
• Headaches
• Hunger
• Nausea

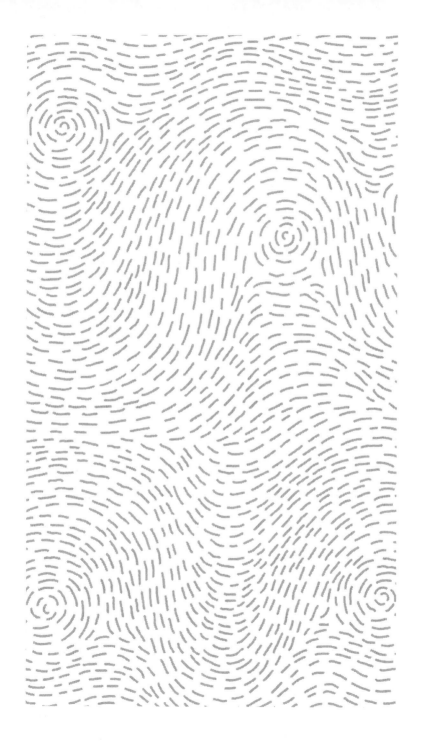

# CHAPTER TWO

# Nature's Pharmacy

Have you ever walked around a bustling farmers' market and marveled at the bounty of glorious fruits and vegetables on display? The mounds of brightly hued produce seem almost magical in their perfection and proliferation. When you take a closer look at the colorful carrots, apples, beets, peppers, and broccoli, it becomes obvious that they are exceptional. These powerful plants are the building blocks of vibrant good health, and they can be key players in successfully banishing disease. Fruits, vegetables, and herbs contain all the vitamins, minerals, amino acids, enzymes, phytochemicals, antioxidants, and phytonutrients your body needs to run efficiently and thrive in today's increasingly polluted world. The question is how to access all that goodness to fuel and heal your body.

Juicing is one way to get the goodness of fruits and vegetables into your body. Juicing bathes your cells, tissues, and organs with powerful nutrients and antioxidants. But it is important to understand exactly what type of natural prescription is in each juice. Each type of fruit, tuber, leaf, flower, stem, and root has different properties with unique strengths. Juicing can take all the bounty in nature's pharmacy and distill it into potent blends that target specific health problems or combinations that sweep out toxins to create a healthier, more efficient body. Becoming familiar with each type of fruit and vegetable is important so you know which natural tools you need in your juicer at any particular time.

## FRUIT JUICE VERSUS VEGETABLE JUICE

Specifically, fruit juices are cleansers and energizers, while vegetable juices are builders and regenerators. Freshly extracted fruit or vegetable juices can supply all the enzymes, vitamins, minerals, protein, and even some fats critical to increased vitality.

### Fabulous Fruits

When you think about your previous experience with juice, before buying your juicer, what was the type of juice you consumed most frequently? If you are like the majority of people, it was probably a fruit juice such as orange or apple. There is certainly nothing wrong with these juices, especially if they are fresh and not prepared with water from concentrate. However, single-source juices or 100 percent fruit juices do not have all the nutrients required for vibrant good health. Fruit provides energy rather than the building blocks to repair and renew.

To state it very simply, the difference between fruit and vegetable juices is the sugar content. Fruit, as a group, is very sweet—almost like eating dessert. Think about lush ripe peaches, dark rich cherries, and sunny juicy oranges. These fruits are delectable, but in some cases too much would make you feel ill because of the sweetness. There are some fruits that are not quite as sweet, but they are usually prepared and used as vegetables, such as tomatoes or winter squash.

Fruit should not be the primary ingredient in the majority of your juice creations. Sometimes a certain health condition requires a predominantly fruit-based juice, but you should avoid consuming only fruit juices. Keep in mind that juicing removes the fiber from the fruit, leaving the sugar content to be absorbed very quickly and converted speedily to energy in the body. This may cause rapidly spiking blood sugar and accompanying headaches, nausea, and dizziness. So use fruit juices as an accent, a flavoring, and a natural sweetener in your vegetable juices. However, don't avoid fruits altogether. They contain valuable nutrients and should be consumed in moderation for your best health.

## Vibrant Vegetables

If you gather up all the vegetables in the farm, or in your local grocery store for that matter, you will be astounded by the proliferation of colors in the vegetable world. There's a veritable rainbow of yellows, reds, greens, oranges, purples, and whites, as well as shades in between. Each color represents a unique and varied combination of nutrients and health benefits, so creating juices using a vast assortment of colors and vegetables is crucial for balance.

Vegetables should be the base of most of your juices because they are the cornerstone of wellness and a healthy body. Use a variety of colors, combined with complementary fruits and herbs, to make exceptional juices that heal and nourish your body.

## HEALING FRUITS

### Apple

This simple fruit is extremely high in antioxidants. In fact, Red Delicious and Granny Smith apples are ranked twelfth and thirteenth in the top one hundred antioxidant-packed foods. Apples add a tart sweetness to most juice combinations, and the tarter the apple, the more malic acid it has, which helps the body detox and increases metabolism.

**Health benefits:** Reduces the risk of certain types of cancer, asthma, and digestive disorders; lowers cholesterol; helps control insulin levels in the blood; detoxifies; promotes heart health.

**Healers:** Apples are low in calories and contain no fat or sodium. They are high in soluble fiber and vitamins A and C. Apples are also a good source of potassium, calcium, iron, phosphorus, and flavonoids.

## Apricot

Apricots are high in antioxidants, which are at maximum potency when the fruit is very ripe. Look for apricots that are slightly soft and a deep orange. Apricots are particularly high in lycopene, which is an antioxidant that inhibits the growth of cancer cells.

**Health benefits:** Protects the eyes by decreasing the risk of cataracts and age-related macular degeneration; reduces the risk of cancer and heart disease.

**Healers:** Apricots are a very good source of beta-carotene and fiber. They are high in magnesium, iron, potassium, and vitamins A, C, and E.

## Avocado

This fruit is a great addition to juices that contain spinach or carrot, because half a fresh avocado can increase the absorption of lycopene and beta-carotene, important carotenoid antioxidants, by 200 to 400 percent. This is because carotenoids are fat soluble and avocados contain monounsaturated fats.

**Health benefits:** Lowers the risk of heart disease and cancer; lowers cholesterol levels; reduces inflammation in the body; promotes liver health.

**Healers:** Despite their green color, avocados are packed with carotenoids such as beta-carotene and lutein. They are high in fiber, folate, oleic acid, omega-3 fatty acids, potassium, and vitamins C and K.

## Banana

This fruit combines perfectly with almost any other vegetable or fruit, providing sweetness and creaminess to juice. Bananas don't "juice" the same way as other fruit, but they may still be used in most juicers, especially if the machine has an attachment for soft fruit.

**Health benefits:** Protects against atherosclerosis, high blood pressure, cancer, and type 2 diabetes; helps improve digestion; reduces acid reflux and heartburn; and boosts mood, because bananas contain tryptophan.

**Healers:** Bananas are a very good source of potassium and very low in sodium. They are high in manganese, fiber, and vitamins $B_6$ and C.

## Blackberry

Blackberries are one of the most nutritious fruits to include in a healthful diet. Use them as soon after purchasing as possible, and wash them well. If you pack blackberries tightly and use the lowest speed on your juicer, the yield from two cups should be about three-quarters of a cup of juice.

**Health benefits:** Protects the immune system; eliminates free radicals, which reduces the risk of heart disease, cancer, diabetes, and macular degeneration; reduces the severity of PMS; promotes a healthy digestive system.

**Healers:** Blackberries are very high in antioxidants, such as ellagic acid, and anthocyanins, which give them their rich dark color. They are a good source of fiber and vitamins C and K.

## Blueberry

These berries are a superfood on any list because they have the highest antioxidant capabilities among vegetables, fruits, and herbs. They should be used as an accent in juices rather than the main ingredient, because it would be incredibly expensive to get a substantial yield of juice.

**Health benefits:** Provides antioxidants, which reduce the risk of cancer, heart disease, diabetes, bladder infections, and cognitive diseases; stabilizes blood sugar; promotes eye health.

**Healers:** Blueberries are packed with phytonutrients, which are antioxidants, and anti-inflammatories. They are very high in folic acid, vitamin C, beta-carotene, calcium, iron, magnesium, potassium, and sodium. They're also a good source of folic acid and vitamins $B_1$, $B_2$, and $B_6$.

## Cantaloupe

One sunny, sweet melon can produce as much as half a gallon of juice. If you want a less sweet, more nutritious juice, cut the skin off your melon, leaving as much green rind as possible, and juice the rind as well.

**Health benefits:** Protects against cancer, macular degeneration, arteriosclerosis, and metabolic syndrome; improves insulin resistance; reduces the risk of diabetes; boosts the metabolism.

**Healers:** Cantaloupe are very high in beta-carotene and vitamins A and C. They're also a good source of potassium, folate, fiber, and vitamins $B_3$, $B_6$, and K.

## Cherry

This lush fruit is quite expensive, so it should be used as a rich accent in juices. Buy the darkest fruit possible to get the highest level of antioxidants.

**Health benefits:** Provides high antioxidant levels, which are effective for treating gout and the pain associated with arthritis; reduces the risk of cancer; fights against urinary tract infections.

**Healers:** Cherries are high in beta-carotene, folic acid, B vitamins, and vitamins C and E. They are also a good source of calcium, magnesium, zinc, iron, and potassium.

## Cranberry

Cranberries are very tart and are best mixed with sweeter fruits or vegetables for palatable juices. Fresh cranberries may be hard to find, except in the winter, so use frozen the rest of the year; they do not lose nutrients when frozen.

**Health benefits:** Treats and prevents urinary tract infections; reduces the risk of kidney stones and prostate cancer.

**Healers:** Cranberries are high in beta-carotene, folic acid, B vitamins, and vitamins C and K. They are a good source of calcium, magnesium, iodine, potassium, and quinine.

## Fig

Figs are a very effective laxative, so it is best to not use too many in any recipe. They do add an intense sweetness to juice. Figs are very perishable, so try to use them within a couple days of buying them.

**Health benefits:** Lowers bad (LDL) cholesterol and blood sugar; strengthens bones; improves digestion; lowers the risk of hypertension.

**Healers:** Figs are a good source of vitamin $B_6$, potassium, calcium, iron, and magnesium. They are also high in pectin.

## Grape

Juicing grapes is easy because you can put both the fruit and stems into your juicer. Grapes are very high in antioxidants, including resveratrol, and if you want a super dose, use black, purple, or red grapes, because their level of antioxidants is higher.

**Health benefits:** Lowers cholesterol and blood pressure; reduces the risk of clots; curbs cognitive decline.

**Healers:** Grapes are very high in folate, beta-carotene, manganese, and vitamins A, $B_1$, $B_2$, $B_6$, C, and E. They are also a good source of vitamin K, calcium, potassium, pectin, and iron.

## Grapefruit

Go for the pink varieties because they contain higher amounts of antioxidants than other types of grapefruits. When preparing your grapefruits for juicing, simply remove a thin layer of the outside peel, leaving as much pith as possible. People who are taking statin medications to lower cholesterol and drugs to control hypertension should not consume grapefruit in any form.

**Health benefits:** Reduces the risk of cancers, such as colon and lung cancer; reduces the risk of osteoporosis; stimulates the digestion; cleanses the lymphatic system.

**Healers:** Grapefruits are an excellent source of vitamins A and C, beta-carotene, and D-glucaric acid. They are a good source of calcium, potassium, thiamine, phosphorous, sodium, pectin, and folate.

## Honeydew

The juice of this bright green melon is best consumed within twenty-four hours of juicing, because it loses its flavor quickly. To prepare it, remove just a thin layer of the skin, leaving the rind, and juice it seeds and all.

**Health benefits:** Boosts the immune system; reduces the risk of heart disease, several cancers, and Alzheimer's disease; protects against cataracts and macular degeneration.

**Healers:** Honeydews are an excellent source of B vitamins, vitamins A and C, and potassium. They are also a good source of vitamin E, folic acid, potassium, copper, zinc, iron, magnesium, and calcium.

## Kiwi

Kiwi is one of the few fruits that is green when it is completely ripe—and it contains chlorophyll. Juice your kiwis when they are very ripe or they may be tart. You may juice the skin if you clean it very carefully and it is not too thick.

**Health benefits:** Protects against and improves respiratory disease; reduces the risk of cancer; detoxifies the body.

**Healers:** Kiwis are an excellent source of potassium, folate, beta-carotene, and vitamins C and K. They are also high in vitamin E, calcium, phosphorus, magnesium, copper, iron, zinc, and omega-3 fatty acids.

## Lemon and Lime

These are quite different fruits but have similar properties and uses in juicing. It is best to leave some white pith on your lemons and limes, because the pith contains high concentrations of a phytochemical called limonene. Add a small amount of lemon or lime juice to intensify the flavor of your vegetable juices.

**Health benefits:** Cleanses and detoxifies the body; reduces the risk of several types of cancers and gallstones.

**Healers:** Lemons and limes are excellent sources of vitamin C and limonene. They are high in potassium, vitamin A, folate, beta-carotene, zinc, magnesium, citric acid, and calcium.

## Mango

Mangoes are high in antioxidants and add a piney sweet taste to juices. Mangoes that are too ripe do not juice well. It is best to use fruit that gives just a little to the touch. Peel them before juicing and slice the mango flesh away from the pit.

**Health benefits:** Boosts the immune system; cleanses the body; reduces the risk of cancer and heart disease.

**Healers:** Mangoes are high in vitamins A and C, beta-carotene, potassium, and niacin. They are a good source of quercetin, calcium, iron, gallic acid, and zinc.

## Nectarine

Nectarines should always be peeled and pitted before juicing. The skin contains bitter oils that may irritate the stomach, and the pit contains amygdalin, which converts to cyanide in the stomach. Let your nectarines ripen at room temperature before using them for juice, so they become sweet.

**Health benefits:** Reduces the risk of cancer; lowers cholesterol; helps regulate blood pressure; reduces the risk of cardiovascular disease.

**Healers:** Nectarines are high in potassium, beta-carotene, and pectin. They are also a good source of calcium, magnesium, iron, zinc, copper, B vitamins, and vitamins A, C, and K.

## Orange

Oranges are incredible combined with other ingredients or juiced alone. Keep the pith on the orange, because it is packed with nutrients. If you suffer from heartburn, you might want to avoid pure orange juice, because the high acid content may aggravate the condition.

**Health benefits:** Combats the common cold; boosts immunity; reduces the risk of cancer; lowers cholesterol.

**Healers:** Oranges are very high in vitamin C and limonoid. They are also a great source of vitamin A, potassium, folate, calcium, iron, and B vitamins.

## Papaya

Papayas have nutrients in all parts (flesh, skin, and seeds), but the skin and seeds may create bitter juice, and you will need a powerful juicer to handle the seeds. Try not to juice the fruit when it is too ripe, because the yield will not be very good.

**Health benefits:** Reduces the risk of cancer, heart disease, eye diseases, and some infections; promotes healthy digestion; improves hay fever and male fertility.

**Healers:** Papayas are high in vitamins A and C, beta-carotene, and potassium. They are also a good source of calcium, iron, magnesium, folate, and proteolytic enzymes.

## Passion Fruit

Passion fruit comes in different colors that have different nutrition profiles. The yellow passion fruit is the most nutritious and contains beta-carotene. Passion fruit is wonderful in blends, because its strong flavor may mask any bitter or unpleasant flavors of the other ingredients.

**Health benefits:** Reduces the risk of cancer, arthritis, and heart disease; promotes healthy digestion and strong bones; lowers blood pressure.

**Healers:** Passion fruits are high in beta-carotene, riboflavin, copper, and vitamins A, $B_2$, and C.

## Peach

Peaches that seem not quite ripe enough are great for juicing. Juice the skin along with the flesh to access all the nutrients, but be sure to remove the pit. Peaches are a great choice when you're trying to lose weight.

**Health benefits:** Helps prevent heart disease, diabetes, cancer, and macular degeneration; boosts immunity; cleanses the kidneys and bladder; promotes good digestion.

**Healers:** Peaches are an excellent source of vitamins A and C, lutein, lycopene, beta-carotene, and folic acid. They are also a good source of calcium, magnesium, zinc, iron, phosphorus, potassium, and niacin.

## Pear

Pears contain a fruit sugar called levulose that people with diabetes can tolerate better than other sugars. You may juice every part of the pear—simply wash it well and remove the stem!

**Health benefits:** Helps detoxify the body; lowers cholesterol; alleviates constipation; reduces the risk of cancer, diabetes, and neurological disorders.

**Healers:** Pears are high in pectin and vitamins $B_6$ and C. They are a good source of copper, potassium, vitamin E, and riboflavin.

## Pineapple

Pineapple combines very well with fruit and vegetable ingredients, providing a rich, sweet taste to recipes. You may juice the core of the pineapple along with the flesh, but it is a good idea to slice off the thick skin unless you have a powerful juicer.

**Health benefits:** Helps reduce excess mucus, which improves asthma and hay fever symptoms; fights the common cold; and improves digestive problems.

**Healers:** Pineapples are high in vitamin C, bromelain, and manganese. They are also a good source of copper, calcium, thiamin, folic acid, potassium, iron, and vitamins $B_6$ and E.

## Plum

Plums can be green, yellow, purple, black, or red. The sweetness of the plum depends on the color, the black and yellow being the sweetest. Plums are very high in antioxidants, which are found in the flesh and skin.

**Health benefits:** Reduces the risk of cancer, heart disease, high blood pressure, cataracts, and macular degeneration; boosts immunity; improves iron absorption; aids digestion; and prevents osteoporosis.

**Healers:** Plums are high in B vitamins and vitamins A and C. They are a good source of pectin, vitamin K, potassium, calcium, and niacin.

## Pumpkin

Pumpkins are packed with nutrients and are a superfood with many health benefits. The best juicing pumpkins are small and sweet. You need to peel and remove the seeds before juicing the flesh. Pumpkin may be enhanced with spices, lemon juice, and fresh ginger.

**Health benefits:** Helps prevent cancer, kidney stones, heart disease, stroke, and ulcers; promotes a healthy digestive system; boosts immunity; reduces cholesterol; helps cure insomnia.

**Healers:** Pumpkins are an excellent source of beta-carotene, B vitamins, and vitamin C and D. They are also high in copper, iron, vitamin E, potassium, and phosphorus.

## Raspberry

Raspberries are packed with antioxidants, and only a handful of raspberries provides an intense flavor to recipes and a healthful dose of nutrients. One cup of fresh berries produces about one-quarter cup of juice.

**Health benefits:** Reduces the risk of heart disease, liver fibrosis, Parkinson's disease, and cancer; boosts the immune system; reduces the signs of aging; promotes healthy skin.

**Healers:** Raspberries are high in manganese, B vitamins, and vitamins C and K. They are also a good source of vitamin E, beta-carotene, niacin, calcium, zinc, potassium, and ellagic acid.

## Strawberry

Ripe strawberries are one of the most popular fruits in the world and also one of the most nutritious. They do not lose a single nutrient when juiced because the entire berry, including the stems, may be put in your juicer. Simply wash them well and juice.

**Health benefits:** Reduces the risk of many cancers, heart disease, and cognitive decline; boosts the immune system; lowers cholesterol and blood pressure; improves digestion; helps stabilize blood sugar.

**Healers:** Strawberries are high in ellagic acid, potassium, beta-carotene, and vitamins A and C. They are also a great source of vitamin E, manganese, folic acid, B vitamins, iron, zinc, and copper.

## Tangerine

Tangerines are a great choice for people who have digestive problems with oranges, because they are less acidic and have more sugar. The skin should always be removed before juicing because it is difficult to digest, but the pith and seeds are quite nutritious.

**Health benefits:** Prevents skin and breast cancer; improves eye health; increases iron absorption; purifies blood; strengthens blood vessels.

**Healers:** Tangerines are high in beta-carotene, potassium, folate, lutein, and vitamins A and C. They are a good source of calcium, magnesium, zinc, and vitamins $B_1$ and $B_2$.

## Tomato

Tomatoes are often used like a vegetable in cooking, but they are in fact a fruit. They combine very well with both vegetable and fruit in juices, and should not be overripe. Do not ever juice green tomatoes, because the resulting juice may irritate the kidneys.

**Health benefits:** Reduces the risk of cancer, heart disease, kidney disease, and hypertension; decreases high blood pressure; cleanses the liver.

**Healers:** Tomatoes are an excellent source of lycopene, potassium, and vitamins A and C. They are a good source of B vitamins, vitamin K, calcium, magnesium, iron, oxalic acid, malic acid, and phosphorus.

## Watermelon

The flesh of watermelon is over 90 percent water, and approximately 95 percent of its nutrition is found in the rind. The best way to juice a watermelon is to peel off the hard outer skin, leaving as much white rind as possible. The rind will make the juice less sweet. Always use watermelon juice right away, because the taste deteriorates after three to five hours.

**Health benefits:** Reduces the risk of heart disease and cancer, especially lung, prostate, and stomach cancers; works as an effective diuretic; promotes a healthy digestive system.

**Healers:** Watermelons are high in lycopene, beta-carotene, and vitamins A and C. They are also a great source of potassium, magnesium, zinc, and vitamins $B_1$ and $B_6$.

## HEALING VEGETABLES

### Asparagus

This slender vegetable creates juice with a strong flavor, so you need only a few spears in any recipe. Juicing is a good way to use thicker, woodier asparagus because you don't have to trim off the tougher parts before adding the spears to the juicer.

**Health benefits:** Detoxifies the body; purifies the blood; reduces the risk of cancer, heart disease, diabetes, and anemia; improves kidney disorders; alleviates arthritis pain; reduces the risk of birth defects.

**Healers:** Asparagus is high in B vitamins, beta-carotene, potassium, manganese, fiber, calcium, iron, and vitamins A, C, E, and K. It is a good source of protein, pantothenic acid, copper, magnesium, and zinc.

## Beet

This sweet vegetable is a very powerful ingredient for juicing. Simply wash the skin of the root and the greens, and then juice everything together for a luscious beverage with a deep color. Beets come in a range of colors, from white to deep ruby red, so experiment to see which you like best.

**Health benefits:** Supports detoxification of the liver; strengthens the gallbladder; supports eye health; reduces the risk of cancer and heart disease; lowers blood pressure; treats anemia by helping to rebuild red blood cells.

**Healers:** Beets are an excellent source of beta-carotene, folate, and vitamins A and C. They are a good source of betaine, potassium, iron, phosphorus, and magnesium.

## Bell Pepper

All the bell peppers—green, yellow, orange, and red—may be used for juicing. Each color has different phytonutrients, and the deeper the color, the higher the concentration of antioxidants. Peppers are sweet and may be juiced with their seeds.

**Health benefits:** Detoxifies the body; reduces the risk of cancer, stroke, heart disease, and blood clots; lowers cholesterol; prevents digestive disorders, macular degeneration, cataracts, and asthma; boosts the immune system.

**Healers:** Bell peppers are high in B vitamins, potassium, and vitamins A, C, and E. They are also rich in magnesium, zinc, calcium, phosphorus, manganese, and silica.

## Bok Choy

This is a generally mild-tasting member of the cabbage family, but the bigger and older the bok choy, the greater its bite. It needs to be washed thoroughly, especially at the bottom where the stems are joined, to remove dirt and avoid gritty juice.

**Health benefits:** Reduces the risk of cancer; lowers cholesterol; promotes healthy brain function, healthy eyes, and bone health; decreases premenstrual symptoms; boosts the immune system.

**Healers:** Bok choy is an excellent source of calcium, vitamin C, potassium, and folate. It is also a good source of vitamins A and K.

## Broccoli

Broccoli is most well known nutritionally for its cancer-fighting abilities. The Hippocrates Institute recommends daily doses of broccoli to prevent cancer, because this vegetable is packed with powerful phytochemicals that protect the body. Make sure your broccoli has no yellow spots, because this means it is not as nutritious, and always include the stems in your juice.

**Health benefits:** Reduces the risk of cancer, heart disease, stroke, and cataracts; boosts the immune system; supports healthy bones and teeth.

**Healers:** Broccoli is high in B vitamins, beta-carotene, calcium, iron, indoles, potassium, sulforaphane, and vitamins A and C. It is a good source of sulfur and the essential amino acids arginine, leucine, lysine, and valine.

## Brussels Sprout

This is one of the most nutritious vegetables in the world, but many people do not like them in juice. It is best to mix Brussels sprouts with other ingredients because the juice does not taste great on its own. Try to get vibrant green heads with no yellowing or soft spots, and juice the entire sprout after washing it thoroughly.

**Health benefits:** Prevents macular degeneration and cataracts; reduces the risk of cancer and heart disease by preventing damage by free radicals in the body; promotes good bone health; stabilizes blood sugar; supports weight loss.

**Healers:** Brussels sprouts are high in iron, potassium, and vitamins A and C. They are a good source of B vitamins, vitamins E and K, and manganese.

## Butternut Squash

This winter squash is technically a fruit because of its seeds. It may be challenging to juice but worth the effort. Remove the skin with a peeler, seed your squash, and cut it into long, thin strips instead of chunks. Butternut squash juice is a glorious sunny color and blends very well with sweet fruit and a touch of spice or ginger.

**Health benefits:** Stabilizes blood sugar; boosts the immune system; reduces the risk of heart disease and cancer; and protects against diabetes, cataracts, macular degeneration, asthma, and rheumatoid arthritis.

**Healers:** Butternut squash is high in beta-carotene, potassium, and vitamins A, $B_6$, C, and E.

## Cabbage

Cabbage is a very strong-tasting vegetable, so it should not be a surprise that the juice is also strong and slightly bitter. It is a healthful addition when mixed with other ingredients, but it may sometimes cause intestinal gas if consumed alone.

**Health benefits:** Improves digestive problems; lowers cholesterol; protects against cancer and heart disease; treats peptic ulcers; detoxifies the body; improves the symptoms of arthritis; reduces the signs of aging.

**Healers:** Cabbage is high in B vitamins, vitamins C and K, and manganese. It is rich in selenium, calcium, potassium, iron, magnesium, and phosphorus.

## Carrot

Carrots are a wonderful healthful base for many juices, both vegetable and fruit, because they are sweet and vibrant. Carrots actually become even more nutritious when you juice them because the nutrients are more available to the body in liquid form. Sweet and vibrant carrots blend equally well with fruits or vegetables.

**Health benefits:** Reduces the risk of cancer and heart disease; improves eye health; boosts the immune system; reduces cholesterol.

**Healers:** Carrots are high in vitamins A and C, beta-carotene, alpha-carotene, lutein, and calcium. They are a good source of vitamins E and K, iron, zinc, potassium, magnesium, and phosphorus.

## Cauliflower

Cauliflower does not yield much juice, but is so nutrient-packed that it should be a staple in your juice-making regimen. This cruciferous vegetable comes in many colors, not just the typical white supermarket kind. Look for bright orange, green, and purple cauliflower at a farmers' market or organic grocer. To extract the maximum amount of juice from cauliflower, use a masticating juicer.

**Health benefits:** Prevents inflammation, arthritis, and osteoporosis; reduces the risk of cancer and heart disease; detoxifies the body; promotes a healthy digestive system; improves the immune system; stabilizes blood sugar.

**Healers:** Cauliflower is high in vitamins C and K, B vitamins, choline, potassium, and fiber. It is also rich in manganese, calcium, magnesium, phosphorus, protein, copper, and iron.

## Celery

Celery is a great addition to vegetable juices because it adds a slightly salty taste, and its mild flavor combines well with other ingredients.

When using a centrifugal juicer, add celery and its greens last. The fibrous strings may clog the basket.

**Health benefits:** Reduces the intensity and frequency of migraines; protects against cardiovascular disease, aching muscles, and neurological diseases; reduces blood pressure and the risk of cancer; detoxifies the body.

**Healers:** Celery is an excellent source of vitamins A and C, B vitamins, sodium, and coumarin. It is also a good source of potassium, calcium, sulfur, silicon, and iron.

## Collard Greens

Collard greens are sometimes a second choice after kale, but they yield more juice and are less expensive than their cousins. Collard greens are best combined with other ingredients, because they are slightly bitter and it would take about eight packed cups to get a glass of juice.

**Health benefits:** Promotes healthy bones and vision; boosts the immune system; reduces the risk of cardiovascular disease, Alzheimer's disease, and cancer.

**Healers:** Collard greens are high in beta-carotene, B vitamins, and vitamins A, C, and K. They are also a good source of calcium, lutein, lipoic acid, and magnesium.

## Cucumber

Cucumbers are a perfect addition to most blends, because they yield an incredible amount of cool, refreshing juice and are very nutritious. Simply rinse off your cucumbers and juice them with the skin and seeds, because most of the nutrition is found in the skin.

**Health benefits:** Acts as a powerful diuretic; reduces the signs of aging; promotes healthy complexion, hair, and nails; reduces inflammation in the body and blood pressure; lowers cholesterol levels.

**Healers:** Cucumbers are an excellent source of silicon, vitamins A and C, and beta-carotene. They are also rich in potassium, manganese, magnesium, vitamin K, phosphorus, and calcium.

## Endive

The endive family includes chicory and escarole. They are sometimes thought to be a lettuce, but they are actually related to daisies. Endive yields a very concentrated juice, so use it to make up one-quarter of your glass of juice or less. It may also be quite bitter, but it is packed with nutrients, so don't avoid this healthful addition to your diet.

**Health benefits:** Promotes eye health and healthy skin; reduces the frequency of asthma attacks; reduces the risk of cancer and anemia; cleanses the body; promotes good digestive health.

**Healers:** Endives are an excellent source of vitamins A and C and calcium. They are also rich in phosphorus, iron, sodium, chlorine, magnesium, potassium, and vitamin $B_1$.

## Fennel

Fennel has a licorice-like taste that may overpower other ingredients and may take a bit of time to get used to. The entire bulb and the feathery fronds may be juiced. It is lovely combined with ginger or Asian pear.

**Health benefits:** Reduces the risk of cancer and heart disease; promotes a healthy digestive system; reduces the symptoms associated with menopause; combats depression.

**Healers:** Fennel is high in vitamin C, potassium, manganese, iron, and B vitamins. It is a good source of magnesium, phosphorus, copper, vitamin E, and zinc.

## Garlic

Garlic is a superfood that has been used for centuries to heal the body. It is best to put just one or two garlic cloves into a glass of juice, because raw garlic can be quite sharp and pungent.

**Health benefits:** Supports a healthy cardiovascular system by lowering cholesterol and blood pressure, and reducing the risk of blood clots; boosts immunity; reduces the risk of cancer; detoxifies the body; stabilizes blood sugar.

**Healers:** Garlic is high in vitamins A and $B_6$, allicin, iron, and potassium. It also contains amino acids and twelve antioxidants, and it is rich in calcium, vitamin C, phosphorus, copper, selenium, and manganese.

## Jicama

Jicama is a crisp, juicy member of the potato family that produces a mild, thick juice. Scrub the skin and juice the entire vegetable without peeling it to retain all the nutrients found just under the skin.

**Health benefits:** Reduces the symptoms of asthma; prevents the flu and colds; boosts the immune system; enhances the complexion; supports weight loss.

**Healers:** Jicama is high in vitamins A and C, B vitamins, and calcium. It is a good source of vitamin K, sodium, potassium, iron, magnesium, phosphorus, manganese, and zinc.

## Kale

Kale produces a deep-green, nutrient-packed juice that combines very well with other ingredients, especially lemon, which intensifies the taste. Kale leaves are quite tough and may sometimes be hard to push through a juicer.

**Health benefits:** Reduces the risk of cancer, type 2 diabetes, heart disease, and stroke; promotes healthy eyesight; increases testosterone; boosts the immune system; and supports the digestive system.

**Healers:** Kale is an excellent source of vitamins A and C, calcium, beta-carotene, alpha-linoleic acid, and chlorophyll. It is a good source of potassium, phosphorus, iron, manganese, copper, magnesium, and B vitamins.

## Lemongrass

Lemongrass is a common ingredient in Asian cuisine. It blends beautifully with other ingredients, especially carrots and ginger. Lemongrass juices best in a masticating juicer because it is quite fibrous.

**Health benefits:** Reduces the risk of cancer, anemia, and diabetes; supports a healthy digestive tract; lowers blood pressure and cholesterol levels; purifies the blood; relieves the symptoms of arthritis, gout, urinary tract infections, heartburn, and colds.

**Healers:** Lemongrass is an excellent source of vitamins A and C, folate, iron, and magnesium. It is rich in B vitamins, calcium, zinc, copper, potassium, phosphorus, and manganese.

## Lettuce

Though lettuce is composed almost entirely of water, it is still a healthful addition to any diet. There are many types of lettuce, and each has a different nutritional profile. The best lettuces for juicing are the ones with darker leaves, such as romaine, red leaf, and green leaf. Wash lettuce thoroughly, one leaf at a time, then juice the entire head, even the core.

**Health benefits:** Reduces the risk of cancer and osteoporosis; detoxifies the body; builds up hemoglobin in the blood; promotes healthy skin and hair; reduces asthma symptoms; cleanses the colon; combats insomnia.

**Healers:** Lettuce is high in chlorophyll, beta-carotene, vitamins A and C, iron, and magnesium. It is a good source of potassium, vitamin K, calcium, phosphorous, B vitamins, copper, and calcium.

## Onion

Onions produce a potent, pungent juice that is wonderful added to vegetable juices. You don't have to peel your onions; simply juice them whole. Juice onions before adding other ingredients. The other vegetables will then clean the lingering onion oils out of the juicer.

**Health benefits:** Reduces the risk of blood clots, diabetes, cancer, heart disease, and anemia; lowers cholesterol and blood pressure; relieves symptoms of arthritis and constipation; boosts immunity; fights the common cold.

**Healers:** Onions are high in organosulfur and vitamins A and $B_6$. They are a very good source of vitamin C, calcium, potassium, phosphorus, magnesium, chromium, and iron.

## Parsnip

Parsnips produce a sweet, milky juice that should be mixed with other juices to tame the taste. Juice these vegetables with the skin on to get all the nutrients.

**Health benefits:** Reduces blood pressure; supports healthy skin and eyes; reduces the symptoms of asthma and arthritis; promotes healthy liver function; reduces the risk of ulcers.

**Healers:** Parsnip is high in folic acid, vitamin K, calcium, and manganese. It is a good source of vitamin C, phosphorus, potassium, and sulfur.

## Pea

Peas are nutritional powerhouses that may be juiced pod and all. Make sure your peas aren't too full and fat, or the juice yield will be scant. If you want to use just the peas for another recipe, juice the pods; they produce a fair amount of juice on their own.

**Health benefits:** Reduces the risk of diabetes, heart disease, cancer, and arthritis; prevents osteoporosis, Alzheimer's disease, insulin resistance, and digestive disorders.

**Healers:** Peas are very high in manganese, phosphorus, B vitamins, and vitamins A, C, and K. They are a good source of protein, magnesium, copper, iron, potassium, and zinc.

## Radish

Radishes add a heat component to juices, ranging from just a slight peppery taste to searing heat, depending on the individual radish. It is best to taste the radishes before adding them to a recipe to gauge their heat contribution. Juice the entire radish after washing it: greens, stem, and flesh.

**Health benefits:** Detoxifies the body; promotes liver, bladder, and gallbladder health; relieves digestive problems and sore throats; reduces the risk of kidney stones, cancer, and asthma.

**Healers:** Radishes are an excellent source of vitamins A and C, B vitamins, potassium, phosphorus, and calcium. They are a good source of copper, zinc, and manganese.

## Sweet Potato

Sweet potatoes are not really potatoes; they are a different type of tuber. They add a sweetness and depth to juices, and are wonderful in fruit combinations. You may juice the skin if you scrub the sweet potatoes well.

**Health benefits:** Boosts the immune system; reduces the risk of cancer and heart disease; promotes a healthy digestive system and complexion; stabilizes blood sugar; fights arthritis, asthma, and the effects of stress.

**Healers:** Sweet potatoes are high in vitamin A, beta-carotene, and chlorogenic acid. They are a good source of calcium, vitamins C and E, potassium, iron, folic acid, and copper.

## Spinach

Spinach is a superfood that may be added to almost any juice recipe with great results—although it might make some juices turn brown. Wash your spinach even if it comes prewashed, and pick through the leaves to remove any slimy ones, which can wreck the juice.

**Health benefits:** Reduces the risk of cancer, macular degeneration, and high blood pressure; cleanses the liver; relieves digestive problems; reduces the pain of arthritis; promotes healing.

**Healers:** Spinach is high in beta-carotene, lutein, protein, iron, and vitamins A, C, and E. It is also a good source of calcium, choline, potassium, magnesium, phosphorus, and folic acid.

## Swiss Chard

This dark, leafy green is beautiful in appearance, and packed with almost every nutrient possible. Chard should be added in moderation to your juicing recipes at least three to four times a week. Look for smaller leaves if you want a less bitter juice, and try all the different colors of stalks—white, yellow, green, orange, and deep red.

**Health benefits:** Stabilizes blood sugar; reduces the risk of macular degeneration, cataracts, cancer, and osteoporosis; promotes healthy skin and hair; boosts immunity.

**Healers:** Swiss chard is high in vitamins A and C, beta-carotene, potassium, iron, calcium, manganese, B vitamins, copper, and phosphorus. It is also a good source of magnesium, zinc, and vitamin E.

## Turnip

Turnips may be an acquired taste, and should probably be combined with other juices because of their strong taste. You may juice both the root and leaves, after washing them thoroughly.

**Health benefits:** Reduces cancer risk, cardiovascular diseases, diabetes, cataracts, asthma, and hypertension; relieves the symptoms of arthritis; promotes digestive health; detoxifies the body.

**Healers:** Turnips are high in vitamin C, calcium, magnesium, lutein, folate, and potassium. They are a good source of phosphorus and iron.

## Wheatgrass

Wheatgrass is an incredibly nutritious food, but it should not be used regularly in juicing because it may cause nausea and is a strong detoxifier. Wheatgrass is quite bitter, so combine small amounts with other juices. It is best to use a masticating juicer with this ingredient.

**Health benefits:** Detoxifies the blood; boosts the immune system and metabolism; improves thyroid function; reduces the risk of osteoporosis; rebuilds red blood cells; promotes a healthy digestive system.

**Healers:** Wheatgrass is an excellent source of chlorophyll, vitamins A and C, B vitamins, calcium, alpha-carotene, and beta-carotene. It is a good source of vitamins E and K, iron, potassium, magnesium, phosphorus, copper, manganese, and zinc.

## Zucchini

Zucchini is a great juice ingredient. It is about 95 percent water, and its mild taste combines well in many recipes. Make sure you get smaller zucchini, because the larger ones may be bitter.

**Health benefits:** Cleanses and detoxifies the body; reduces the risk of cancer, diabetes, stroke, heart disease, kidney disease, arthritis, and gout; promotes a healthy digestive system and skin; boosts the metabolism; lowers cholesterol and blood sugar.

**Healers:** Zucchini is high in vitamins C and K, B vitamins, potassium, and magnesium. It is a good source of vitamin A, copper, phosphorus, calcium, protein, zinc, and beta-carotene.

## THE TOXIC TWENTY

Vegetables and fruits are a crucial part of a nutritious diet, and the whole idea behind juicing is to get all the nutrients from your produce that contribute to good health and vitality. So the very last thing you want are pesticides piggybacking on your produce. Pesticides are present in some amount on most commercially grown produce. Often the pesticides are found on the skin. Unfortunately, you do not want to peel your produce in most cases because there are many nutrients found in and just under the skin. Washing your produce won't remove all the pesticide residue, either, but it may help a little.

There is not enough research to show exactly what impact pesticide exposure at the levels found on produce will ultimately have on people. But we certainly know that pesticides are dangerous chemicals—which is why their use is highly regulated. Pesticide exposure is thought to cause:

- Birth defects
- Brain tumors
- Cancer
- Childhood leukemia
- Fertility problems
- Hormone and endocrine system problems
- Nervous system damage
- Non-Hodgkin's lymphoma

**The U.S. Department of Agriculture tested forty-eight popular fruit and vegetable crops for pesticides.** They found that 67 percent of this produce had at least one kind of pesticide residue, and 11 percent of the tested produce had five or more pesticides.

There are certain fruits and vegetables that you should always strive to source from organic growers; these types of produce are deemed by the Environmental Working Group to be the most contaminated by pesticides. This non-profit organization puts out a shopping guide every year that lists the pesticide load in forty-five types of produce, pinpointing the ones that are the most contaminated (the "toxic twenty"), as well as the "Capsicum," which are the least contaminated. Buying this usually contaminated produce from certified organic suppliers may cut your exposure to dangerous pesticides by as much as 90 percent. The toxic twenty are:

1. Apples
2. Strawberries
3. Grapes
4. Celery
5. Peaches
6. Spinach
7. Sweet bell peppers
8. Nectarines (imported)
9. Cucumbers
10. Potatoes
11. Cherry tomatoes
12. Hot peppers
13. Blueberries (domestic)
14. Lettuce
15. Snap peas (imported)
16. Kale / collard greens
17. Cherries
18. Nectarines (domestic)
19. Pears
20. Plums

It is not realistic to try to ensure that every fruit, vegetable, and herb you use in your juicing recipes will be organic, because you might not have access to organic options for every type of produce. Plus, organic produce may be expensive. Just try to limit your exposure to pesticides and other additives so that juicing provides the healing power and nutrition you are looking for in your diet. Always wash your ingredients thoroughly and store them safely before juicing.

## HEALING ADD-INS

Making delicious juices is all about combining different fruits and vegetables in the right amounts. Herbs and spices may also be added to juices to create truly delicious drinks. Many add-ins also add their own benefits to your healthful juice.

### Allspice

Allspice is a pungent, warm spice that adds dimension to any juice recipe. It is a great addition to pumpkin, apple, butternut squash, and pear juices.

**Health benefits:** Relieves symptoms associated with digestive problems, arthritis, and premenstrual syndrome; reduces the risk of diabetes, high blood pressure, and obesity.

**Healers:** Allspice is high in vitamin C, calcium, manganese, iron, and magnesium. It is a good source of copper, phosphorus, potassium, zinc, and selenium.

### Basil

Basil is one of the most popular herbs in the world because of its fragrance and wonderful flavor. Basil is a perfect addition to juices because it has antibacterial properties that diminish the presence of an infectious bacteria found on raw produce. This means your juices will be safer to drink

**Health benefits:** Supports cardiovascular health; reduces the severity of symptoms of inflammatory bowel syndrome, asthma, rheumatoid arthritis, and osteoarthritis.

**Healers:** Basil is high in vitamins A and K, iron, and calcium. It is a good source of manganese, tryptophan, vitamins $B_6$ and C, magnesium, and potassium.

## Cayenne Pepper

Cayenne is a member of the *Capsicum* family, a relative of bell peppers. The fresh cayenne peppers are dried and then ground up into powder. These peppers contain capsaicin, which is responsible for the hotness of the powder. Just a pinch of cayenne can spice up any juice recipe.

**Health benefits:** Reduces the risk of diabetes, stroke, heart disease, and stomach ulcers; lowers cholesterol; boosts immunity; decreases the symptoms of asthma, cluster headaches, osteoarthritis, and rheumatoid arthritis.

**Healers:** Cayenne is an excellent source of beta-carotene and vitamins A, $B_6$, C, and E. It is a good source of vitamin K and manganese.

. . . . . . . . . . . . . . . . . . . . . . . . . . . . . . . . . . . . . . . . . . . . . . . .

**Once you master various fruit, vegetable, and add-in blends, there are other ingredients you may add to your juices for flavor, texture, and health benefits.** If you want something different, try adding olive oil, ginseng, apple cider vinegar, hemp seed, wheat germ, coconut oil, spirulina, or honey.

. . . . . . . . . . . . . . . . . . . . . . . . . . . . . . . . . . . . . . . . . . . . . . . .

## Cilantro

Cilantro leaves have a bright, pungent, unique flavor that is used in Asian and South American cooking. Juice the whole plant—leaves and stems. Cilantro is very different from coriander, which is the seed of the same plant, and they cannot be substituted for each other in recipes.

**Health benefits:** Cleanses toxic metals from the body; reduces the risk of diabetes, cardiovascular disease, and osteoporosis; lowers blood sugar and cholesterol levels; promotes healthy vision and skin.

**Healers:** Cilantro is an excellent source of vitamins A, C, and K. It is rich in manganese, folate, iron, vitamin $B_6$, potassium, calcium, and magnesium.

## Cinnamon

Ground cinnamon is made from the bark of the related cinnamon or cassia trees, and it adds a warm, fragrant, sweet taste to juices. The intense healing provided by cinnamon comes from the components in the essential oils of the bark, called cinnamaldehyde, cinnamyl acetate, and cinnamyl alcohol.

**Health benefits:** Lowers the risk of blood clots and heart disease; helps normalize blood sugar; boosts brain activity; lowers cholesterol; promotes a healthy digestive tract.

**Healers:** Cinnamon is high in vitamin K, iron, manganese, and calcium. It is a good source of iron, magnesium, phosphorus, potassium, copper, and vitamins $B_6$, C, and E.

## Cloves

Anyone who has been to the dentist will recognize the taste of cloves, which is used as an antibacterial agent during procedures. Cloves are the flower buds of the clove tree, an evergreen. Cloves have a warm, fragrant flavor.

**Health benefits:** Provides very strong anti-inflammatory properties, which benefit the whole body; reduces the risk of cancer and joint inflammation; protects against environmental toxins.

**Healers:** Cloves are high in manganese, omega-3 fatty acids, and vitamin K. They are a good source of vitamin C, magnesium, and calcium.

## Cumin

Cumin seeds have a strong peppery, citrusy, nutty flavor that combines well with many other ingredients.

**Health benefits:** Promotes a healthy digestive system; boosts the immune system and metabolism; reduces the risk of cancer, improves the oxygen-carrying capacity of hemoglobin.

**Healers:** Cumin is high in iron. It is a good source of manganese, calcium, and magnesium.

## Ginger

Ginger is the rhizome from the ginger plant. It has been used for centuries as a remedy for gastrointestinal distress, but it also has other benefits—along with a lovely, pungent, spicy flavor.

**Health benefits:** Alleviates nausea associated with sea sickness, morning sickness, and motion sickness; lessens the pain of osteoarthritis and rheumatoid arthritis; boosts immunity; reduces the risk of cancer.

**Healers:** Ginger is high in magnesium, potassium, manganese, copper, and vitamins $B_6$ and C. It is a good source of calcium, iron, phosphorus, and zinc.

## Mint

Mint has a distinctive cool flavor that comes from a component called menthol. This herb is incredible combined with melon, cucumber, or apples. Juice the whole plant—leaves and stems.

**Health benefits:** Promotes liver health; stimulates digestion; reduces nausea; boosts immunity; fights colds and flu; reduces the risk of cancer; cleanses the blood.

**Healers:** Mint is high in vitamins A and C. It is a good source of calcium, copper, vitamin $B_2$, manganese, iron, potassium, and magnesium.

## Mustard Seed

Mustard seeds add a spicy taste to juices and are delicious with carrots and parsnips. Do not substitute mustard powder for the seeds, because the flavor will not be as strong.

**Health benefits:** Reduces the risk of cancer, heart attack, and migraines; lowers blood pressure; reduces the symptoms of rheumatoid arthritis, menopause, and asthma.

**Healers:** Mustard seeds are an excellent source of selenium. They are a good source of manganese, omega-3 fatty acids, magnesium, and phosphorus.

## Parsley

This herb is usually used for garnish and often left on the plate, but it enhances the healing properties of any juice recipe. Make sure you wash parsley well. Soak it in a bowl full of water, rinsing several times to remove all dirt and grit. Juice the whole plant—leaves and stems.

**Health benefits:** Reduces the risk of cancer, heart attack, stroke, atherosclerosis, diabetes, and asthma; boosts the immune system; purifies the blood; promotes eye health.

**Healers:** Parsley is an excellent source of chlorophyll, beta-carotene, and vitamins A, C, and K. It is a good source of folate, magnesium, iron, calcium, manganese, potassium, and zinc.

## Rosemary

Rosemary is known for its heady fragrance and has a long healing history. You don't need very much of this herb to flavor any juice recipe. If your rosemary has tough, woody stems, strip the leaves off into the juicer, but if the stems are supple, you may juice them as well.

**Health benefits:** Detoxifies the liver; boosts mood and memory; provides relief from pain associated with headaches and arthritis; reduces the risk of cancer; improves digestion and blood circulation; promotes a healthy immune system.

**Healers:** Rosemary is a good source of calcium, iron, and vitamins: A, $B_6$, and C.

## Sage

Sage is very high in antioxidants and should be a regular choice for juicing. It has a strong fragrance and flavor, so only use a couple of leaves at first and build up to more if you enjoy the taste. Juice the whole plant—leaves and stems.

**Health benefits:** Promotes healthy bones; reduces the risk of cancer; improves blood clotting; decreases inflammation; promotes increased brain function; reduces the risk of Alzheimer's disease, asthma, and cardiovascular disease.

**Healers:** Sage is an excellent source of vitamin K, calcium, and potassium. It is a good source of beta-carotene.

## Thyme

A delicate herb with a clean, sharp fragrance, thyme is an addition to most classic French and Mediterranean cuisines. It also complements almost any fruit and vegetable you might want to add to juicing recipes. Thyme is very high in flavonoids and healthful volatile oils. Juice the whole plant—leaves and stems.

**Health benefits:** Promotes a healthy digestive system; relieves respiratory conditions and arthritis; boosts immunity; detoxifies the liver.

**Healers:** Thyme is rich in vitamin K, iron, manganese, calcium, and potassium. It is a good source of magnesium and vitamins A, B6, C, and E.

## Turmeric

This peppery, warm spice will make your juices a sunny yellow color. The taste is similar to a perfect melding of orange and ginger. Turmeric is a rhizome, but it is found almost exclusively in powdered form.

**Health benefits:** Reduces the risk of cancer, Alzheimer's disease, and heart disease; promotes healthy liver function; stabilizes blood sugar; lowers cholesterol; helps relieve Crohn's disease, colitis, and rheumatoid arthritis.

**Healers:** Turmeric is a good source of manganese, vitamin B6, iron, and potassium.

## POTENT COMBINATIONS

Every fruit, vegetable, herb, and spice has an individual nutritional profile that can benefit the body in some way. Sometimes, combining certain types of produce—and thus combining their benefits—in a juice recipe targets specific health problems and diseases. The nutrients, antioxidants, and phytochemicals complement one another and strengthen the effect on the body. If you are trying to specifically relieve or prevent a physical ailment or condition, it may be valuable to create juices using ingredients that are particularly potent together. Some powerful health benefits provided by combinations are:

- **Acne:** Carrot, mango, pumpkin
- **Alzheimer's disease:** Broccoli, carrot, onion, spinach
- **Anemia:** Beet, lemon, strawberry, Swiss chard
- **Anti-aging:** Apple, avocado, cabbage, cranberry
- **Arthritis:** Carrot, celery, cucumber, pineapple
- **Asthma:** Bell pepper, carrot, pear
- **Bone health:** Kiwi, parsley, spinach
- **Cancer:** Blackberry, broccoli, kale, pumpkin
- **Constipation:** Beet, Brussels sprout, grape, pumpkin
- **Digestive problems:** Apple, fennel, peach, spinach
- **Fatigue:** Apricot, cantaloupe, parsnip, spinach
- **Halitosis:** Apple, fennel, lime, spinach
- **Heart disease:** Broccoli, garlic, parsley, tomato
- **High blood pressure:** Cabbage, celery, garlic, lemon
- **High cholesterol:** Blueberry, carrot, orange, Swiss chard

## SEVEN TIPS FOR MAKING GREAT JUICES

The definition of a great juice may vary, depending on your priorities and what you want to get out of juicing. You could be looking to relieve or prevent a certain health problem or to simply improve your overall health. If you are targeting a disease, a great juice might be one that combines vitamins, phytonutrients, and antioxidants for maximum effect in the body. Or a great juice could be one that tastes like summer in a glass and is the perfect vehicle to make sure your kids get their daily servings of fruits and vegetables. Whatever your definition of great is, there are some strategies you can use to get the most out of juicing.

1. **Start with high-quality ingredients.** Your finished juice is going to be only as good as the fruit, vegetables, and herbs you put in your juicer. Make sure the ingredients are fresh, unspoiled, and not bruised. You do not have to buy organic products, but it is a good idea whenever possible, especially when using any of the toxic twenty. Organic fruits and vegetables often taste better because they are naturally ripened, so the flavor develops perfectly.

2. **Drink your juice right away.** When fresh juice sits around exposed to air, it loses nutrients and the health benefits of drinking it are diminished. It also tastes the best fresh out of the juicer! Sometimes it is not convenient or economical to juice for only immediate use, especially when you're doing a juice cleanse. If you do juice a large batch, store the extra juice in airtight jars in the refrigerator or freezer. When freezing juices, make sure you account for the fact that liquids expand when they freeze, and leave some space at the top of the jar.

3. **Combine different flavors.** Juices are best when they have some complexity, created by blending different tastes rather than having only one or even two flavors in the glass. Try to meld tart, sweet, and herbaceous. Don't avoid ingredients that might be bitter or earthy, like kale or arugula; instead, balance them out with other flavors. Also include a fruit or vegetable that yields a fair amount of juice, such as cucumber, as a nice mild base. This ensures that the juice is not too potent to drink.

4. **Juice your favorite produce combinations.** When thinking about the types of ingredients you are going to use for juicing, think of your favorite combinations in salads or soups. For example, a rich, fresh gazpacho or your preferred salad has ingredients that you can also juice together. Keep in mind that you might have to tinker with the quantities of the ingredients and add a high-yield item such as celery to bulk up the results.

5. **Start your juicing experiments slowly.** When you first get your juicer, stick with fruits and vegetables you are familiar with and those whose juice you might have tried before, such as carrot, apple, or cucumber. Don't jump right in and juice an entire head of kale or even spinach— you might never fire up the juicer again from the flavor shock! Earthy or bitter greens should be combined in small amounts with sweeter or milder-tasting produce until you are used to the potent results coming out of the juicer.

6. **Refine and enhance your juices.** If you are going to pick one or two ingredients to have in almost every juice you make, the best choice is ginger or lemon (or both). Lemon has the ability to brighten or sharpen the flavor of other ingredients, creating a superior juice. Ginger has a similar flavor-heightening effect in small quantities. Make sure you don't use too much of either, or the flavors of the other ingredients in the juice will be overwhelmed.

7. **Don't be afraid of vegetables.** Think about the store-bought juice combinations you already may drink. You'll likely come up with an assortment of fruit-based creations, with the occasional addition of tomato (also a fruit) or carrot. These ingredients are sweet and pleasing to the palate, so it makes sense that they would dominate the commercial juice landscape. However, when making juices at home, it is best to expand your palate. Make sure to include more vegetables than fruits to avoid overdosing on natural sugar. Vegetable juices are fresh and satisfying with loads of nutrients, and a hint of sweetness from a well-placed mango or handful of berries can make them sublime.

# CHAPTER THREE

# Juice Cleansing for Health

Any juicing is a positive step toward better health, so simply adding a fresh juice twice or three times a week to your diet can make a huge difference physically and mentally. The question you will eventually ask yourself, after juicing starts to make you feel strong and vibrant, is what you would feel like after a complete cleanse. The answer to that can be found only by trying a cleanse yourself.

Keep in mind that beginning a detox or cleanse on the spur of the moment, with no thought to your end goals and no real plan, is highly inadvisable. You can't simply cut out all food and fire up your juicer for every meal—at least not without getting sick, which is the opposite outcome you are seeking with a juice cleanse. Conveniently, you're reading this book, and this chapter will help you safely and effectively plan juice cleanses.

## WHAT IS A JUICE CLEANSE?

In today's technology-driven, pollution-plagued world, there are toxins everywhere. They are in the air, the water, and even in the foods we eat to nourish our bodies. Someone who eats only organic foods and minimizes their exposure to harmful chemicals will still have some contamination in their body. We all breathe the air around us, after all.

Even the normal processes in the body produce waste that needs to be flushed out for continued good health. Clearing out the accumulated toxins and organic debris cluttering up your body's systems can contribute to healthier, more efficient organs and processes within the body. This accumulation of toxins starts at birth; toxins settle in the fat and organs, creating health problems such as nutritional deficiencies, hormone imbalances, and poor metabolism and immune function.

Perhaps you have tried adding juicing once a day or once every few days, and the results have been very positive. Now you want to really experience the full power of juicing and the associated benefits of cleansing your entire body. It may be confusing to get started with this type of change, and the last thing you want to do is jump in uninformed. You may be asking:

- Why would someone want to do a juice cleanse?
- What exactly is a cleanse?
- Is it the same as fasting or detoxing?

## Juice Cleansing

A juice cleanse is when you drink a predominantly juice-based diet for several days to gently cleanse your body of toxins system-wide. You may eat a small amount of solid foods during a juice cleanse, but it is more effective if your intake of solid food is limited. Typically, during a juice cleanse you drink only fresh juices and herbal teas for at least one day and up to three days.

If you do decide to do a juice cleanse, don't starve yourself. The idea behind cleansing is to heal and clean the body, not to lose weight. Make sure your calorie, nutrient, protein, and fat intake supports your body's needs. This means at least 2,000 calories per day and a very broad range of juices to ensure you get a variety of nutrients. A juice cleanse may be done once a week, once a month, or whenever you want to cleanse your body to maintain good health.

## Detoxing

A detox is a much more intense undertaking that is done to cleanse the body more deeply or target specific organs or toxins in the body. Detoxing is usually done for at least a week and sometimes longer, depending on your commitment and the level of contamination in your body. It is extremely important to consult your doctor before beginning a juice detox, because it could do more harm than good, depending on your physical state.

A detox is about rebooting your metabolism or starting fresh after ending unhealthful life choices. It should never be a maintenance routine you do all the time to try to counterbalance unhealthful eating habits.

## Fasting

Fasting usually means abstaining from food entirely and consuming only water. This is not an ideal choice for people who need to continue working and doing all their activities. Fasting may be beneficial, but only after you are used to doing detoxes and have a relatively light toxin burden in the body. You may do a juice fast, which is not as severe because you are drinking fresh juices as well as water. Juice fasts are usually short and are almost identical to detoxing.

## BENEFITS OF A CLEANSE

Juicing fruits and vegetables is a wonderful way to add nutrients to your diet, and the health benefits of a juice cleanse are far-reaching. The benefits vary depending on the level of toxin contamination you have in the body and whether you are specifically targeting an organ, such as the liver or colon. There are many benefits that may be achieved through a cleanse, including:

- Balanced pH
- Better digestion
- Better kidney function
- Better sense of taste and smell
- Better sleep
- Blood cleansing
- Colon cleansing
- Decreased, healthier appetite
- Diminished allergies
- Glowing complexion
- Healthier nails and hair
- Improved cardiovascular health
- Improved fertility and more regular menstrual cycle
- Improved liver function
- Increased energy levels
- Increased mental clarity
- Less chronic pain
- Less cravings for sugar or caffeine
- Less heavy metals in the body
- Lowered toxin load in the body
- Reduced bloating and water retention
- Reset metabolism
- Regular bowel movements
- Sense of well-being
- Stable blood sugar levels
- Stronger immune system
- Weight loss

During a cleanse, the fresh juices and water you drink should provide your body with everything it needs, including electrolytes, nutrients, salt, enzymes, and energy. You should not feel unwell during a cleanse or really hungry, because there are enough calories in fresh juices to keep you satisfied. If you find you are reacting badly to a longer cleanse, rather than experiencing the benefits, discontinue it until you consult a doctor. Or try to build up to a longer cleanse through a succession of one-day cleanses.

## IS A CLEANSE RIGHT FOR YOU?

Juice cleanses are not appropriate for everyone, and should never be done without consulting a doctor even if you do not fall within the list of people for whom they are not recommended. Even if it is not recommended to do a full juice cleanse because of an existing circumstance or health condition, you may still include healthful juices as a supplement to a regular nutritious diet. Juice cleanses should not be done if you have/are:

- An eating disorder or past history of one
- An impaired immune system
- Cancer
- Diabetes
- Epilepsy
- Kidney disease
- Liver disease
- Low blood pressure
- Stomach ulcers
- Malnourished
- Pregnant or nursing
- Undergoing chemotherapy

If you take medication for an existing health condition, you need to talk to your doctor about the ramifications of undertaking a juice cleanse. Many medications indicate on the label that they must be taken with food. These types of medication need fiber and digestive activity to distribute and release the medicine. If you have the slightest question or doubt, talk to your doctor.

If you are unable to do a juice cleanse and you are still concerned about toxin build-up in your body, you can always make diet changes that also remove toxins. Some changes to consider are eliminating alcohol, processed foods, excess sugar, saturated fats, and white flour. Eat a diet packed with whole grains, healthful lean meat or no meat, and an abundant assortment of fruits and vegetables. And, of course, add fresh juices to your diet.

## TIPS FOR A SAFE AND SUCCESSFUL CLEANSE

Juice cleanses are a bit of a trend right now, and some people are tempted to simply jump in and start juicing, and cleansing, without any goal or preparation. This is not the path to success. Cleanses can be truly uplifting, physically beneficial processes if done correctly, with plenty of thought and planning. Here are some tips to help you get through your juice cleanse successfully and safely.

**Consult your doctor.** You've heard this before, and it's worth hearing again. The relationship between food and the body is incredibly powerful and intricately balanced. Doing anything different, especially a juice cleanse, which is quite a dramatic change, may have unforeseen consequences. Your current physical state, diet, level of activity, and toxin contamination all come into play when doing a juice cleanse. So make an appointment and discuss your plans with your doctor to see what personal stumbling blocks might be in your way and what advice you get from a professional.

**Start small (or short in this case).** Don't jump right into a week or more of detox without first trying a day or two or three. It is a good strategy to do several shorter cleanses to get your body accustomed to the process and give you an idea of what to expect from a longer, more intense cleanse.

**One small eight-ounce glass of juice per day can double your consumption of nutrients.** Your intake of minerals, vitamins, enzymes, and antioxidants all go up by over 100 percent. Imagine what a 100 percent juice cleanse adds to your system!

**Make some healthful changes in the week before the cleanse.** Make the transition to consuming just juice easier by acclimatizing your body. This will make withdrawals from certain foods easier and your juicing experience more pleasant. Some changes to consider are:

- Cut back on your sodium intake.
- Cut back on your sugar consumption.
- Don't overindulge in fatty foods.
- Drink plenty of water.
- Include more raw vegetables and fruits in your diet.
- Stop drinking alcohol and smoking.
- Stop drinking coffee.

**Prepare and do your research.** Look into juice cleanses thoroughly (such as reading this book) before starting a cleanse. Figure out what kind of cleanse you want to do. You may target specific organs, such as the liver, colon, or kidneys, or do an overall body cleanse, depending on your needs.

**Tell close friends and family of your plan.** You certainly don't have to tell everyone what you are doing, but it is a good idea to inform those closest to you so they can offer support. This can ensure you don't unintentionally get tempted to go off your cleanse by someone who does not know your goal. It might also be a good idea not to plan too many social activities during your cleanse to avoid situations that are centered on food and alcohol.

**Plan your juices.** It is always better to have a specific game plan and the resources you need available when committing to a big change like a juice cleanse. This will also save you money, because you can shop for everything you need at the same time.

**Don't limit your juice intake.** You should make sure you get enough calories and schedule your juices regularly throughout the day, so that you don't experience plummeting blood sugar and a loss of energy.

**Make a variety of juices.** A good mix of different vegetables and fruits, as well as herbs and spices, makes your cleanse interesting and fun. Try to plan your juices to be about 80 percent vegetables so you don't end up consuming too much sugar from fruit. Some specific conditions require fruit juices to get the right blend of nutrients, but don't use pounds of fruit in all your blends.

**Don't exercise too much.** If you are a world-class athlete or just extremely active before starting your juice cleanse, you may continue working out. You might experience a drop in energy, but that is normal. Instead of intense workouts, try walking, yoga, or a nice leisurely bike ride to get physical.

**If you are a beginner at juice cleansing, you might feel nauseous the first day or two of the cleanse.** Your body will not be used to the potent, concentrated flavor and nutritional impact of the juice. Try diluting your juices at a one-to-one ratio with water until you feel fine. If you have no problem with the potency of the juices, make sure you drink as much water as you do juice during the cleanse. This will ensure your system is hydrated enough to flush out the toxins.

**Quit if you react badly.** Since the goal of a juice cleanse is to get healthier and feel better, it makes no sense to continue a cleanse if you feel truly horrible or experience severe physical symptoms. Feeling fatigued, a bit headachy, and nauseous is normal, and may have more to do with withdrawal from caffeine or sugar and dehydration. These symptoms will pass. However, if you feel very ill, stop the cleanse and consult your doctor.

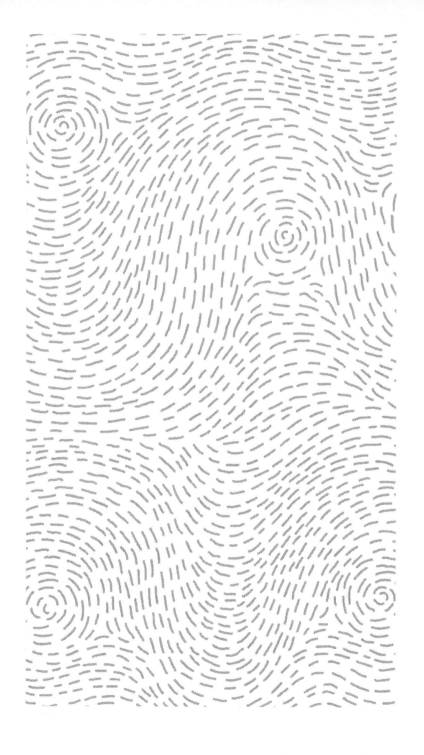

# CHAPTER FOUR

# Juicing Cleanse and Detox Plans

The cleanse and detox plans in this chapter are guidelines—a framework to get you started—so you can try a cleanse with no guesswork. You do not have to follow them exactly, especially if one of the recipes does not appeal to you. If you want to substitute another recipe from this book, that's is fine. You may even create your own targeted recipes using the "make your own" suggestions following each recipe. If you don't like an ingredient in a recipe, collard greens for example, substitute a similar ingredient, such as spinach or kale, so the recipe still maintains its texture and intent.

Once you decide to try a three-day cleanse or a longer seven-day detox, it is important to prepare yourself with these five steps so that you have the best chance for success.

1. Pick a time in your schedule when you can do your cleanse without too many (or any) outside events or activities. One reason for this is so you can concentrate on your body and mentally detox as well. The other reason you may want to clear out a little time is you could experience some physical reactions to your cleanse, such as loose bowel movements, cramps, or headaches. Having some time to yourself while this is going on might be the best strategy.

2. At least a couple weeks before your start date, cut back on or quit caffeine, alcohol, and cigarettes, so the effects you feel on your cleanse aren't withdrawal symptoms from these habits.

3. At least a week before your cleanse, cut out or substantially decrease your intake of processed foods, dairy, meat, gluten, and saturated fats. Pay close attention to refined sugars, because sugar cravings may completely derail your cleanse if your body has not become accustomed to being without sugar.

4. A week before your cleanse, start eating a predominantly vegan diet, so your body gets used to loads of fresh fruit and vegetables.

5. Get enough sleep the night before you do a cleanse, so you are bright-eyed and ready to go in the morning.

**A juice cleanse might be a good time to detox mentally as well as physically.** Try meditation to clear your head, and if you find your motivation wavering, concentrate on the reasons you wanted to detox in the first place. Detoxing may cause anxiety because it is a huge change for your body, so find something relaxing to do instead of stressing yourself needlessly about your cleanse.

Even if you have been preparing for your cleanse, it will still probably be challenging to do even a three-day juice cleanse because people are creatures of habit. Eating solid food at regular intervals is a lifetime habit, so feelings of deprivation will be normal even if your body is not really missing food. Here are some detoxing strategies to ensure a successful cleanse or detox challenge.

• Choose a variety of different juices so you stay interested and your body gets a full range of nutrients. Shoot for every possible color of fruits and vegetables during each day.

• Try to use organic produce, if possible, to avoid adding any new toxins to your body during your cleanse.

- Drink lots and lots of water to facilitate the flushing of your system. Try to drink one to two glasses of water (preferably filtered water) after each glass of juice, and stay hydrated at all times.
- Don't be surprised if you feel a little ill the first day as your body starts to cleanse itself. Headaches, nausea, bad breath, and dizziness are quite normal.
- Slow down on your exercise routine during your cleanse. Choose walks and yoga instead of spinning and running.
- Start the day with a glass of warm water combined with the juice from half a lemon to get your digestive tract moving. This does not count as one of your meals, just a preparation.
- If you are doing the seven-day challenge, you might want to shop for your ingredients in two trips: one just before you start and one midweek, so that everything is fresh.

The three-day juice cleanse and seven-day detox challenge will have you drinking five or six 16- to 20-ounce juices each day. This volume is about double what a usual juice portion would be to ensure that you get enough calories to maintain your body. These plans use juices found in Part Two of this book. The serving sizes in the recipes are usually 8 to 12 ounces, so when you are following the cleanse and detox plans, simply double the serving size for each meal.

## THREE-DAY PURE JUICE CLEANSE PLAN

Over the three-day cleanse, you will be drinking five different types of juice per day. The plan is designed to be approximately 2,000 calories a day and cover a full spectrum of nutrients. This is a pure juice cleanse, which means you will not be eating solid food for the entire three days. You may have as much herbal tea (unsweetened) and water as you wish, along with the juices.

······························································

**Did you know that drinking lemon juice in warm water can stimulate the gastrointestinal tract, and lemons help keep your body alkaline?** Lemons are usually thought to be acidic, and this is true outside the body. When inside the body, they are alkaline and people who eat a more alkaline diet lose weight quicker than those who consume an acidic diet.

······························································

Make sure you "chew" your juices rather than simply pouring them down. Chewing starts the digestive process by mixing an enzyme from your mouth called ptyalin into your juice, which helps to break the food down—even juices—and start the digestive process. Chewing also gives the juice time to match the temperature of your body, so it is immediately accessible when you do swallow.

## Day One

**WHEN YOU RISE**   12 OUNCES OF WARM WATER MIXED WITH THE JUICE FROM HALF A LEMON

**BREAKFAST**   LDL REDUCER

**MIDMORNING**   BEET THE HEAT

**LUNCH**   CLEAN ARTERY SWEEP

**MIDAFTERNOON**   SHINY TRESSES

**DINNER**   SWEET DREAMS

**BEFORE BED**   AN HERBAL TEA OF YOUR CHOICE

## Day Two

**WHEN YOU RISE**   12 OUNCES OF WARM WATER MIXED WITH THE JUICE FROM HALF A LEMON

**BREAKFAST**   DOES A BODY GOOD

**MIDMORNING**  CARROT COLON CLEANSE

**LUNCH**  GREAT GRAPEFRUIT CLEANSE

**MIDAFTERNOON**  FOCUS ON HYDRATION

**DINNER**  HEART BEET

**BEFORE BED**  AN HERBAL TEA OF YOUR CHOICE


## Day Three

**WHEN YOU RISE**  12 OUNCES OF WARM WATER MIXED WITH THE
JUICE FROM HALF A LEMON

**BREAKFAST**  CLEAN AS A WHISTLE KIDNEY CLEANSE

**MIDMORNING**  GARDEN FRESH BLAST

**LUNCH**  LDL REDUCER

**MIDAFTERNOON**  BURN, BABY, BURN

**DINNER**  SPINACH SUGAR STABILIZER

**BEFORE BED**  AN HERBAL TEA OF YOUR CHOICE


## SEVEN-DAY DETOX CHALLENGE

Over the seven-day detox, you will be drinking five different types of juice per day. The diet is designed to be approximately 2,000 calories a day and cover a full spectrum of nutrients. This is a pure juice detox, which means you will not be eating solid food for the entire week. If you feel you need to eat something, stick to a salad made entirely of raw foods, so you don't counteract everything you are trying to achieve by detoxing. You may have as much herbal tea (unsweetened) and water as you wish, along with the juices.

After your detox is complete, ease back into regular food rather than eating an enormous meal. Stick with light meals and juices for the first few days until your body adjusts to solid food again.

## Day One

**WHEN YOU RISE**  12 OUNCES OF WARM WATER MIXED WITH THE JUICE FROM HALF A LEMON

**BREAKFAST**  DOES A BODY GOOD

**MIDMORNING**  BEET THE HEAT

**LUNCH**  CLEAN ARTERY SWEEP

**MIDAFTERNOON**  SHINY TRESSES

**DINNER**  SWEET DREAMS

**BEFORE BED**  AN HERBAL TEA OF YOUR CHOICE

## Day Two

**WHEN YOU RISE**  12 OUNCES OF WARM WATER MIXED WITH THE JUICE FROM HALF A LEMON

**BREAKFAST**  LDL REDUCER

**MIDMORNING**  CARROT COLON CLEANSE

**LUNCH**  FOCUS ON HYDRATION

**MIDAFTERNOON**  HEART BEET

**DINNER**  GARDEN FRESH BLAST

**BEFORE BED**  AN HERBAL TEA OF YOUR CHOICE

## Day Three

**WHEN YOU RISE**  12 OUNCES OF WARM WATER MIXED WITH THE JUICE FROM HALF A LEMON

**BREAKFAST**  GREAT GRAPEFRUIT CLEANSE

**MIDMORNING**  HAPPY COLON

**LUNCH**  SIMPLY WHEATGRASS

**MIDAFTERNOON**   BURN, BABY, BURN

**DINNER**   LDL REDUCER

**BEFORE BED**   AN HERBAL TEA OF YOUR CHOICE


## Day Four

**WHEN YOU RISE**   12 OUNCES OF WARM WATER MIXED WITH THE JUICE FROM HALF A LEMON

**BREAKFAST**   INFLAMMATION BUSTER

**MIDMORNING**   BONNY BONE FRUIT SURPRISE

**LUNCH**   UNDER PRESSURE

**MIDAFTERNOON**   GREEN GO-GO

**DINNER**   LOVE BOOST

**BEFORE BED**   AN HERBAL TEA OF YOUR CHOICE


## Day Five

**WHEN YOU RISE**   12 OUNCES OF WARM WATER MIXED WITH THE JUICE FROM HALF A LEMON

**BREAKFAST**   SPINACH SUGAR STABILIZER

**MIDMORNING**   GET THINGS MOVING

**LUNCH**   GLOWING GINSENG

**MIDAFTERNOON**   PICK ME UP

**DINNER**   ROSY RELAXER

**BEFORE BED**   AN HERBAL TEA OF YOUR CHOICE

## Day Six

**WHEN YOU RISE**   12 OUNCES OF WARM WATER MIXED WITH THE JUICE FROM HALF A LEMON

**BREAKFAST**   CLEAN AS A WHISTLE KIDNEY CLEANSE

**MIDMORNING**   CARROT CLEAR UP

**LUNCH**   HAPPY IN A GLASS

**MIDAFTERNOON**   PASSIONATELY IMMUNE

**DINNER**   BEAT BREAST CANCER

**BEFORE BED**   AN HERBAL TEA OF YOUR CHOICE


## Day Seven

**WHEN YOU RISE**   12 OUNCES OF WARM WATER MIXED WITH THE JUICE FROM HALF A LEMON

**BREAKFAST**   LDL REDUCER

**MIDMORNING**   CITRUS CELLULITE BE GONE

**LUNCH**   HEALTHFUL HEART GINGER

**MIDAFTERNOON**   READY TO RECOVER

**DINNER**   GUT FLORA BUILDER

**BEFORE BED**   AN HERBAL TEA OF YOUR CHOICE

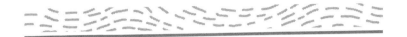

PART TWO

# Recipes for Health

**CHAPTER FIVE:** GENERAL HEALTH AND WELL-BEING

**CHAPTER SIX:** IMMUNE SYSTEM SUPPORT

**CHAPTER SEVEN:** WEIGHT LOSS AND DIGESTION ENHANCERS

**CHAPTER EIGHT:** CANCER AND DISEASE PREVENTION

**CHAPTER NINE:** ENERGY AND VITALITY BOOST

**CHAPTER TEN:** TAMING INFLAMMATION

**CHAPTER ELEVEN:** MIND, BRAIN, AND MENTAL WELLNESS

**CHAPTER TWELVE:** BEAUTY AND SKIN ENHANCERS

This is where you put everything you have learned about juicing, plus your own creativity, into practice by making delicious, healthful juices. The recipes in this section are divided into categories that pinpoint certain types of health concerns, such as cancer and inflammation. You may make any one of these recipes even if you do not have the health problem it is designed to heal.

Each recipe also gives a yield estimate for the finished juice, but that is just a guideline. The amount of juice produced for any given recipe will depend on the ripeness and size of the produce, whether or not it is organic, and what type of juicer you are using. The nutritional information with each recipe is per serving.

Juicing is all about experimentation, and sometimes you will find a combination of fruit and vegetables that is marvelous while other times the blend won't appeal to you. If you don't like a certain recipe but still wish to target that health concern, try experimenting with the list of choices following each recipe until you have a winner. Enjoy yourself, and happy juicing!

# CHAPTER FIVE

# General Health and Well-Being

ACHY BREAKY MUSCLES

BALANCING ACT

BEET CRAMPS

BEET THE HEAT

BLADDER INFECTION
BE GONE

CARROT COLON CLEANSE

CLEAN AS A WHISTLE
KIDNEY CLEANSE

CLEAN ARTERY SWEEP

GARDEN FRESH BLAST

GREAT GRAPEFRUIT CLEANSE

GREEN JOINT RELIEF

HEART BEET

LDL REDUCER

HEALTHY PROSTATE BLEND

LOVE BOOST

SPINACH SUGAR STABILIZER

STIMULATING SUNSHINE

HEALTHY HEART
SUMMER SALAD

UNDER PRESSURE

# Achy Breaky Muscles

MAKES ABOUT 24 OUNCES, 3 SERVINGS

▶ CALORIES: 64, FAT: 1 G, SUGAR: 13 G, PROTEIN: 2 G,
CARBOHYDRATES: 20 G

*Muscles may become sore due to physical exertion, a fall, or even the flu. Achy Breaky Muscles juice is a great way to alleviate the pain of overworked or injured muscles. Fruits and vegetables high in potassium and vitamins C and E, such as oranges and romaine lettuce, can help repair muscle fiber rupture due to free radicals. Ginger is packed with gingerol, which fights inflammation and helps soothe aching muscles, so if you like your juice spicy, add a little more ginger to this juice.*

2 MEDIUM GRANNY SMITH APPLES

1 HEAD ROMAINE LETTUCE

4 SPRIGS MINT

1 ORANGE

2 LARGE CELERY STALKS

½ LARGE ENGLISH CUCUMBER

ONE ¾-INCH SLICE WATERMELON

ONE 1-INCH PIECE GINGER

Core and cut the apples into quarters. Juice the apples, romaine, and mint. Peel the skin off the orange, leaving the pith, and cut it into wedges. Juice the celery, cucumber, watermelon, orange, and ginger. Stir to blend the juice before drinking.

**INGREDIENTS TO EASE ACHING MUSCLES:**

- Banana
- Blackberry
- Blueberry
- Broccoli
- Celery
- Ginger
- Lemon
- Lime
- Orange
- Pineapple
- Pomegranate
- Raspberry
- Romaine lettuce
- Spinach
- Tart cherry
- Tomato
- Watermelon

# Balancing Act

▶ CALORIES: 100, FAT: 1 G, SUGAR: 17 G, PROTEIN: 4 G, CARBOHYDRATES: 30 G

*Hormone levels in most women are a delicate balancing act that can be thrown off by too much or too little estrogen or progesterone. Most women experience an imbalance that is due to too much estrogen. This type of hormone imbalance can cause PMS and an elevated risk of heart disease, depression, and breast cancer. You can balance your hormones by including at least five servings of fruits and vegetables per day, as in this delicious juice. The best choices include produce with deep colors, such as reds, oranges, yellows, and dark greens. Vitamin C is also a good addition, because this vitamin can increase progesterone production in the body, which balances the estrogen.*

2 LARGE CARROTS
½ LARGE RUBY-RED GRAPEFRUIT
1 MEDIUM BEET WITH GREENS
ONE 1-INCH PIECE GINGER

Cut the ends off the carrots. Peel the grapefruit, leaving the pith, and cut it into chunks. Juice the carrots, beet, ginger, and then the grapefruit. Stir to combine the juice before drinking.

**INGREDIENTS TO HELP BALANCE HORMONES:**

- Beet
- Bell pepper
- Blackberry
- Blueberry
- Bok choy
- Broccoli
- Carrot
- Collard greens
- Kale
- Lemon
- Lime
- Orange
- Raspberry
- Spinach
- Tomato

# Beet Cramps

MAKES ABOUT 16 OUNCES, 2 SERVINGS

▶   CALORIES: 110, FAT: 1 G, SUGAR: 20 G, PROTEIN: 4 G,
    CARBOHYDRATES: 32 G

*Probably half of all women suffer from painful menstrual cramps
due to hormonal changes. Including the right vitamins and minerals
in your diet can significantly reduce the pain of cramps. Some of the
most important nutrients that prevent and treat cramps are zinc and
vitamins $B_6$ and C, which are all found in high amounts in spinach. The
parsley used to flavor this rich juice contains a compound called apiole,
which studies have linked to relief from menstrual cramps.*

4 MEDIUM CARROTS
1 GREEN APPLE
2 SMALL BEETS WITH GREENS
½ ENGLISH CUCUMBER
½ CUP CHOPPED SPINACH
½ CUP PARSLEY
¼ CUP MINT
ONE ½-INCH PIECE GINGER

Cut the ends off the carrots. Core the apple and cut it into quarters.
Juice the carrots, beets, and cucumber. Push the spinach, parsley,
mint, and ginger through the juicer with the apple wedges. Stir to
blend the juice before serving.

## INGREDIENTS TO PREVENT OR EASE MENSTRUAL CRAMPS:

- Apple
- Banana
- Beet
- Broccoli
- Brussels sprout
- Carrot
- Celery
- Kale
- Parsley
- Pineapple
- Spinach
- Sweet potato
- Swiss chard

# Beet the Heat

MAKES ABOUT 32 OUNCES, 4 SERVINGS

▶ CALORIES: 60, FAT: 1 G, SUGAR: 10 G, PROTEIN: 3 G, CARBOHYDRATES: 18 G

*The liver is one of the hardest-working organs in the body. It removes impurities from the blood, converts nutrients from food into usable components, and produces enzymes and proteins, all while helping to balance hormones. Cleansing the liver can ensure that the body works well, and Beet the Heat juice has all the ingredients needed to keep the liver strong. Some important nutrients for liver cleansing include antioxidants, phytochemicals, chlorophyll, and vitamin C found in brightly colored produce. The components in the ingredients of this juice help the liver break down fats and expel them, activate liver enzymes, and generally cleanse and detoxify the liver.*

6 LARGE CARROTS
1 MEDIUM APPLE
2 LARGE CELERY STALKS
2 MEDIUM BEETS WITH GREENS
¼ SMALL JALAPEÑO PEPPER, SEEDS REMOVED
1 BUNCH SPINACH

Cut the ends off the carrots. Core the apple and cut it into wedges. Juice the carrots, celery, beets, and jalapeño pepper. Push the spinach through the juicer with the apple. Stir to combine the juice before drinking.

**INGREDIENTS TO CLEANSE THE LIVER:**

- Apple
- Avocado
- Beet
- Bell pepper
- Bok choy
- Broccoli
- Brussels sprout
- Cabbage
- Carrot
- Cauliflower
- Celery
- Citrus fruit
- Garlic
- Ginger
- Grapefruit
- Jalapeño pepper
- Leek
- Parsnip
- Plum
- Pumpkin
- Radish
- Spinach
- Tomato
- Wheatgrass

# Bladder Infection Be Gone

MAKES ABOUT 16 OUNCES, 2 SERVINGS

▶ CALORIES: 94, FAT: 1 G, SUGAR: 19 G, PROTEIN: 1 G,
CARBOHYDRATES: 27 G

*Urinary tract infections and inflammations are common among women and are usually caused by bacteria. This infection may spread to the bladder and kidneys, causing intense discomfort. It is very important to keep hydrated, so water, along with fresh fruit and vegetable juices, can be the best defense. Cranberries are the first-line fruit to utilize in this particular situation. This is because cranberries contain D-mannose, a simple sugar that binds to bacteria and other infectious agents, and stops them from sticking to the lining of the urinary tract. Fruits and vegetables high in vitamin C (which creates a hostile environment for bacteria in the urine) and vitamin A (which helps boost the immune system) are also great choices to banish these infections.*

TWO 2-INCH SLICES WATERMELON

½ LEMON

1 CUP BLUEBERRIES

2 LARGE CELERY STALKS

½ CUP CRANBERRIES

Cut the outer skin off the watermelon, taking off as little as possible. Peel the lemon, leaving the pith, and cut it in half. Remove any visible seeds. Juice half of the watermelon with the blueberries. Juice the celery, cranberries, and the other half of the watermelon. Juice the lemon. Stir to blend the juice before drinking.

## INGREDIENTS TO PREVENT OR TREAT URINARY TRACT INFECTIONS:

- Asparagus
- Blueberry
- Cranberry
- Grapefruit
- Guava
- Lemon
- Lemongrass
- Lime
- Orange
- Pomegranate
- Pumpkin
- Savoy cabbage
- Spinach
- Tomato
- Watermelon
- Wheatgrass

# Carrot Colon Cleanse

MAKES ABOUT 32 OUNCES, 4 SERVINGS

▶    CALORIES: 75, FAT: 1 G, SUGAR: 14 G, PROTEIN: 3 G,
CARBOHYDRATES: 40 G

*The accumulation of mucus in the colon can be a health problem, so cleansing the colon with fresh juiced vegetables and fruits is a great idea to strengthen the immune system and reduce the risk of colon cancer. This delicious juice uses carrots, which help digestion, and beets, which are a fabulous source of soluble fiber. The pectin in the apples strengthens the intestinal lining and flushes out toxins in the colon. All of these super colon-cleansing ingredients combine to create a wonderful drink that will help your digestion work beautifully.*

3 MEDIUM CARROTS
1 GRANNY SMITH APPLE
1 LEMON
2 MEDIUM BEETS WITH GREENS
2 CUPS BLUEBERRIES
½ CUP BROCCOLI FLORETS
ONE 2-INCH PIECE GINGER

Cut the ends off the carrots. Core the apple and cut it into chunks. Peel the lemon, leaving the pith, and cut it in half. Remove any visible seeds. Juice the carrots, beets, blueberries, apple, broccoli, lemon, and ginger. Stir to blend the juice before drinking.

## INGREDIENTS FOR COLON CLEANSING:

- Apple
- Asparagus
- Avocado
- Beet
- Blueberry
- Brussels sprout
- Cabbage
- Carrot
- Cauliflower
- Celery
- Citrus fruit
- Collard greens
- Fennel
- Pumpkin
- Spinach
- Strawberry
- Swiss chard
- Turnips

# Clean as a Whistle
# Kidney Cleanse

MAKES ABOUT 32 OUNCES, 4 SERVINGS

▶ CALORIES: 65, FAT: 0 G, SUGAR: 13 G, PROTEIN: 1 G,
CARBOHYDRATES: 18 G

*The kidneys remove waste products and excess water from the body by processing about 200 quarts of blood every day. This can leave toxins in the kidneys that need to be flushed out. Cleansing your kidneys not only removes toxins; it can also reduce the risk of kidney stones. Including certain foods in your meals, either raw or in the form of this lovely juice, can help keep your kidneys functioning effectively. Blueberries are packed with antioxidants and can flush uric acid out of the kidneys. Both parsley and watermelon are natural diuretics, so more fluid volume and toxins are flushed out. Make sure you hydrate well when taking in this type of cleansing juice.*

5 CUPS DICED WATERMELON
1 LIME
½ CUP PARSLEY
2 CUPS BLUEBERRIES
DASH OF CAYENNE PEPPER

Remove the outer skin from the watermelon, keeping as much white rind as possible just under the skin. Peel the lime, leaving the pith, and cut it in half. Remove any visible seeds, because they will make the juice bitter. Juice the parsley with the watermelon and blueberries. Juice the lime. Stir the cayenne pepper into the juice before drinking.

**INGREDIENTS FOR KIDNEY CLEANSING:**

- Apple
- Asparagus
- Bell pepper
- Blueberry
- Cauliflower
- Cherry
- Coriander
- Cranberry
- Dandelion greens
- Garlic
- Kale
- Lemon
- Onion
- Parsley
- Pumpkin
- Spinach
- Watercress
- Watermelon

# Clean Artery Sweep

MAKES ABOUT 24 OUNCES, 3 SERVINGS

▶ CALORIES: 71, FAT: 1 G, SUGAR: 9 G, PROTEIN: 4 G,
CARBOHYDRATES: 20 G

*Arteriosclerosis (a buildup of plaque in the arteries that can lead to heart attacks) affects many people, but it can be controlled by a diet low in saturated fats and high in fruits and vegetables. The ingredients in this potent juice are very high in antioxidants, which stop bad (LDL) cholesterol from building up on artery walls.*

5 MEDIUM CARROTS
1 LARGE GRANNY SMITH APPLE
1 LIME
3 LARGE CELERY STALKS
1 LARGE ENGLISH CUCUMBER
1 BROCCOLI STALK
3 KALE LEAVES

Cut the ends off the carrots. Core the apple and cut it into quarters. Peel the lime, leaving the pith, and cut it in half. Remove any visible seeds, because they will make the juice bitter. Juice the carrots, celery, cucumber, apple, and broccoli. Juice the kale with the lime. Stir to combine the juice before drinking.

**INGREDIENTS TO HELP PREVENT ARTERIOSCLEROSIS:**

- Apple
- Apricot
- Banana
- Blueberry
- Broccoli
- Cantaloupe
- Carrot
- Celery
- Citrus fruit
- Collard greens
- Garlic
- Ginger
- Honeydew melon
- Kale
- Mango
- Peach
- Pomegranate
- Raspberry

# Garden Fresh Blast

MAKES ABOUT 32 OUNCES, 3 SERVINGS

▶ CALORIES: 33, FAT: 0 G, SUGAR: 5 G, PROTEIN: 2 G,
CARBOHYDRATES: 10 G

*Anemia results when your body does not have enough red blood cells.
The tomatoes in this recipe provide lovely fresh flavor and are a great
source of vitamin C and iron, which supports the formation of new red
blood cells. The iron in the spinach also builds the blood and supports
the synthesis of hemoglobin.*

2 LARGE CARROTS
1 SMALL RED BELL PEPPER
¼ LEMON
3 LARGE CELERY STALKS
3 MEDIUM TOMATOES
1 CUP CHOPPED SPINACH
½ CUP BASIL
¼ CUP PARSLEY
½ SMALL ENGLISH CUCUMBER
½ SMALL JALAPEÑO PEPPER, SEEDS REMOVED
DASH OF BLACK PEPPER

Cut the ends off the carrots. Remove the stem from the red pepper.
Peel the lemon, leaving the pith, and cut it in half. Remove any visible
seeds. Juice the celery, tomatoes, carrots, and red pepper. Push the
spinach, basil, and parsley through the juicer using the cucumber.
Juice the jalapeño pepper and the lemon. Stir to combine the juice,
and season it with black pepper before drinking.

**INGREDIENTS FOR PREVENTING ANEMIA:**

- Apple
- Apricot
- Avocado
- Blueberry
- Broccoli
- Cantaloupe
- Carrot
- Citrus fruit
- Collard greens
- Garlic
- Ginger
- Grape
- Kale
- Passion fruit
- Peach
- Pomegranate
- Raspberry

# Great Grapefruit Cleanse

MAKES ABOUT 32 OUNCES, 4 SERVINGS

► CALORIES: 89, FAT: 3 G, SUGAR: 11 G, PROTEIN: 2 G,
CARBOHYDRATES: 21 G

*The liver is so important to the body that it deserves a strong cleanse recipe to keep it in top form. The Great Grapefruit Cleanse contains only ingredients that are potent cleansing agents. Besides the high dose of vitamin C, along with the allicin and selenium in the garlic, this recipe also includes flaxseed oil and turmeric, which help flush out toxins and dietary carcinogens.*

6 LARGE LEMONS

3 RUBY-RED GRAPEFRUITS

3 GARLIC CLOVES

ONE 4-INCH PIECE GINGER

2 TEASPOONS FLAXSEED OIL

¼ TEASPOON TURMERIC

FILTERED WATER AS NEEDED

Peel the lemons and grapefruits, leaving the pith, and cut them into quarters. Remove any visible seeds. Peel the garlic cloves. Juice the lemons and 2 of the grapefruits. Juice the ginger, garlic, and remaining grapefruit at the same time. Stir to combine the juice, and then add the flaxseed oil and turmeric. Stir again. Add water if the juice seems too thick. Drink immediately.

**INGREDIENTS FOR LIVER CLEANSING:**

- Apple
- Beet
- Bell pepper
- Bok choy
- Broccoli
- Brussels sprout
- Cabbage
- Carrot
- Cauliflower
- Celery
- Citrus fruit
- Garlic
- Grapefruit
- Jalapeño pepper
- Leek
- Parsnip
- Plum
- Pumpkin
- Spinach
- Wheatgrass

# Green Joint Relief

MAKES ABOUT 24 OUNCES, 3 SERVINGS

▶ CALORIES: 76, FAT: 0 G, SUGAR: 16 G, PROTEIN: 1 G,
CARBOHYDRATES: 24 G

*This is a simple green juice that uses a huge dose of dark, leafy greens to provide relief to sore joints. These ingredients contain powerful anti-inflammatory properties that ease painful joints due to arthritis or simple wear and tear. These choices are alkaline, so they dissolve the buildup of deposits around the joints that can create pain. The pear in this juice helps sweeten the green vegetables and herbs, which can often taste bitter, especially for people new to juicing.*

1 BROCCOLI STALK
1 PEAR
2 CUPS KALE
2 CUPS PARSLEY
ONE 2-INCH PIECE GINGER ROOT

Chop broccoli into florets. Cut the pear in half. Juice the kale and parsley, pushing it through the juicer with the broccoli pieces. Juice the ginger and pear. Stir to combine the juice before drinking.

**INGREDIENTS TO EASE JOINT PAIN:**

- Apple
- Beet
- Bok choy
- Broccoli
- Carrot
- Cauliflower
- Collard greens
- Garlic
- Ginger
- Grape
- Grapefruit

- Kale
- Lettuce
- Parsley
- Passion fruit
- Pear
- Pineapple
- Pomegranate
- Raspberry
- Spinach
- Strawberry

# Heart Beet

▶ CALORIES: 99, FAT: 1 G, SUGAR: 16 G, PROTEIN: 3 G, CARBOHYDRATES: 27 G

*Heart disease is an epidemic in many countries, and eating heart-friendly foods high in phytonutrients is the key to reducing the risk of this disease. Phytonutrients, in particular allicin, quercetin, anthocyanidins, and resveratrol, benefit the heart and protect against damage from free radicals. The fruits and vegetables in Heart Beet juice are packed with lutein, anthocyanin, ellagic acid, vitamin C, folate, calcium, magnesium, potassium, and beta-carotene, as well.*

3 LARGE CARROTS

1 PEAR

4 LARGE CELERY STALKS

1 LARGE BEET, PREFERABLY GOLDEN, WITH GREENS

ONE ½-INCH PIECE GINGER

½ ENGLISH CUCUMBER

Cut the ends off the carrots. Cut the pear in half. Juice the celery, carrots, beet, and pear. Juice the ginger and cucumber. Stir to combine the juice before serving.

**INGREDIENTS FOR HEART HEALTH:**

- Apple
- Apricot
- Asparagus
- Avocado
- Beet
- Bell pepper
- Blueberry
- Broccoli
- Carrot
- Celery
- Cranberry
- Fig
- Garlic
- Grape
- Honeydew melon
- Kale
- Onion
- Orange
- Parsnip
- Raspberry
- Spinach
- Strawberry
- Sweet potato
- Tomato

# LDL Reducer

MAKES ABOUT 20 OUNCES, 2 SERVINGS

▶ CALORIES: 111, FAT: 1 G, SUGAR: 21 G, PROTEIN: 4 G,
CARBOHYDRATES: 35 G

*High cholesterol is one of the major risk factors for cardiovascular
disease, and it can be controlled by good diet choices, including
nourishing juices. Celery contains a chemical called butylphthalide
that reduces bad (LDL) cholesterol. An antioxidant found in apples
called polyphenol also lowers bad cholesterol, so this juice has double
the fighting power.*

1 GREEN APPLE
1 LEMON
6 LARGE CELERY STALKS
½ BUNCH SWISS CHARD
1 ENGLISH CUCUMBER

Core the apple and cut it into quarters. Peel the lemon, leaving the
pith, and cut the lemon into quarters. Remove any visible seeds,
because they will make the juice bitter. Juice the celery and apple.
Push the Swiss chard through the juicer with the cucumber. Juice
the lemon. Stir to combine the juice before drinking.

**INGREDIENTS TO LOWER CHOLESTEROL:**

- Apple
- Banana
- Blackberry
- Blueberry
- Broccoli
- Cabbage
- Carrot
- Collard greens
- Cucumber
- Fig
- Garlic
- Kale
- Kiwi
- Lemongrass
- Nectarine
- Orange
- Papaya
- Parsley
- Pear
- Pumpkin
- Raspberry
- Red grape
- Spinach
- Strawberry
- Tomato
- Watermelon

# Healthy Prostate Blend

MAKES ABOUT 24 OUNCES, 3 SERVINGS

▶ CALORIES: 86, FAT: 2 G, SUGAR: 7 G, PROTEIN: 7 G, CARBOHYDRATES: 28 G

*Prostate cancer is the most common cancer in men and it is very treatable if caught early. Diet choices, including fresh vegetable and fruit juices, are a great way to promote prostate health and cut the risk of prostate cancer. This vegetable-packed juice is high in lycopene, which is linked to reduced tumor growth, and several ingredients are high in vitamin C (broccoli, lemon, and lime), which reduces the risk of developing prostate cancer.*

2 SMALL GRANNY SMITH APPLES

1 LEMON

1 LIME

1 CUP BROCCOLI FLORETS

3 BRUSSELS SPROUTS

2 CUPS CHOPPED SPINACH

1 CUP PARSLEY

1 SMALL ENGLISH CUCUMBER

ONE ½-INCH PIECE GINGER

1 TOMATO

Core the apples and cut them into quarters. Peel the lemon and lime, leaving the pith, and cut them in half. Remove any visible seeds, because they will make the juice bitter. Juice the apples, broccoli, and Brussels sprouts. Push the spinach, parsley, and ginger through the juicer using the cucumber. Juice the tomato, lemon, and lime. Stir to blend the juice.

## INGREDIENTS FOR PROSTATE HEALTH:

- Arugula
- Bell pepper
- Bok choy
- Broccoli
- Brussels sprout
- Carrot
- Cauliflower
- Collard greens
- Guava
- Kale
- Lettuce
- Orange
- Papaya
- Pink grapefruit
- Pomegranate
- Squash
- Tomato
- Watermelon

# Love Boost

MAKES ABOUT 16 OUNCES, 2 SERVINGS

▶ CALORIES: 84, FAT: 1 G, SUGAR: 8 G, PROTEIN: 4 G,
CARBOHYDRATES: 22 G

*Libido can be strongly affected by what you eat, and this refreshing juice contains vitamins, hormones, zinc, and other nutrients that support a healthy sex life for women and men. Vitamin A, found in carrots, stimulates the skin, making it more sensitive. The humble celery stalk contains a hormone called androsterone, and kale is high in zinc—both of which boost sex drive. The combination of all the ingredients, especially cucumber, produces a hydrating juice that also promotes endurance and stamina. So instead of a nice glass of wine during a romantic evening, try a glass of Love Boost.*

4 LARGE CARROTS
3 LARGE CELERY STALKS
½ SMALL ENGLISH CUCUMBER
4 LARGE KALE LEAVES
ONE 1-INCH PIECE GINGER

Cut the ends off the carrots. Juice the carrots, celery, cucumber, kale, and ginger. Stir to blend the juice before drinking.

**INGREDIENTS FOR INCREASED LIBIDO:**

- Avocado
- Blueberry
- Broccoli
- Carrot
- Celery
- Chili pepper
- Clove
- Cucumber
- Fig
- Garlic
- Ginger
- Kale
- Lemon
- Saffron
- Spinach
- Turmeric
- Watermelon

# Spinach Sugar Stabilizer

MAKES ABOUT 16 OUNCES, 2 SERVINGS

▶ CALORIES: 93, FAT: 1 G, SUGAR: 15 G, PROTEIN: 5 G,
CARBOHYDRATES: 27 G

*Problems with high blood sugar can lead to many serious health problems,
such as diabetes, insulin resistance, and metabolic syndrome. Spinach
Sugar Stabilizer juice contains fruits and vegetables that are high in
vitamins A, C, and K, which help stabilize blood sugar. This tasty juice
also features cinnamon, which makes cells more sensitive to insulin, a
hormone that converts the sugar in the blood to energy.*

1 LARGE CARROT
½ GRANNY SMITH APPLE
3 CUPS CHOPPED SPINACH
1 CUP PARSLEY
1 CUP BROCCOLI FLORETS
1 CUCUMBER
½ TEASPOON GROUND CINNAMON

Cut the end off the carrot. Core the apple and cut it into quarters.
Push the spinach and parsley through the juicer with the broccoli.
Juice the carrot, apple, and cucumber. Stir the cinnamon into the
juice before drinking.

## INGREDIENTS TO STABILIZE BLOOD SUGAR:

- Apple
- Broccoli
- Brussels sprout
- Cabbage
- Cantaloupe
- Cinnamon
- Fig
- Garlic
- Leek
- Lemon
- Lime
- Mango
- Okra
- Onion
- Orange
- Romaine lettuce
- Spinach
- Yam

# Stimulating Sunshine

MAKES ABOUT 16 OUNCES, 2 SERVINGS

▶ CALORIES: 62, FAT: 1 G, SUGAR: 7 G, PROTEIN: 3 G, CARBOHYDRATES: 21 G

*Men can use potent, fresh juices to maintain a healthy sex life. It might be surprising to know that diet can affect sexual performance and promote a healthy reproductive system. One of the best combinations for sexual health is produce that is high in lycopene (tomatoes, watermelon, and grapefruit, for instance), juiced with dark, leafy greens like spinach. The fruits and vegetables in this pretty yellow juice are packed with phytonutrients, antioxidants, and vitamins that reduce the risk of enlarged prostate, which can be linked to sexual problems. Combine Stimulating Sunshine juice with regular exercise to ensure good sexual function.*

1 LEMON

1 LIME

1 LARGE ENGLISH CUCUMBER

2 LARGE CELERY STALKS

1 LARGE TOMATO

1 CUP CHOPPED SPINACH

ONE 1-INCH PIECE GINGER

½ TEASPOON TURMERIC

Peel the lemon and lime, leaving the pith, and cut it in half. Remove any visible seeds. Juice the cucumber, celery, and tomato. Juice the spinach by pushing it through the juicer with the lemon, lime, and ginger. Stir the turmeric into the juice before drinking.

**INGREDIENTS TO SUPPORT MALE SEXUAL FUNCTION:**

- Asparagus
- Beet
- Bok choy
- Broccoli
- Brussels sprout
- Cabbage
- Garlic
- Onion
- Red carrot
- Ruby red grapefruit
- Spinach
- Swiss chard
- Tomato
- Watermelon

# Healthy Heart Summer Salad

MAKES ABOUT 24 OUNCES, 3 SERVINGS

▶ CALORIES: 63, FAT: 1 G, SUGAR: 10 G, PROTEIN: 2 G, CARBOHYDRATES: 19 G

*Every ingredient found in this flavor-packed juice can help lower cholesterol levels. Bad (LDL) cholesterol levels are directly affected by diet, especially the amount of fruit and vegetables you choose to eat every day. Vegetables like spinach and beet greens contain lutein, which can stop cholesterol from building up on artery walls. Garlic is a superfood that is linked to heart health because it can lower cholesterol and prevent blood clots.*

5 LARGE CARROTS
1 GREEN APPLE
1 SMALL BEET WITH GREENS
1 GARLIC CLOVE
ONE ½-INCH PIECE GINGER
2 CUPS CHOPPED SPINACH
½ CUP PARSLEY

Cut the ends off the carrots. Core the apple and cut it into quarters. Juice the carrots and beet with the garlic and ginger. Push the spinach and parsley through the juicer with the apple quarters. Stir to combine the juice before drinking.

**INGREDIENTS TO LOWER CHOLESTEROL:**

- Apple
- Asparagus
- Avocado
- Beet
- Blueberry
- Broccoli
- Brussels sprout
- Cabbage
- Fig
- Garlic
- Lemongrass
- Nectarine
- Orange
- Pear
- Pomegranate
- Pumpkin
- Raspberry
- Red bell pepper
- Red grape
- Spinach
- Strawberry

# Under Pressure

▶ CALORIES: 40, FAT: 0 G, SUGAR: 4 G, PROTEIN: 2 G,
CARBOHYDRATES: 16 G

*High blood pressure is the main risk factor associated with stroke
and heart disease, so it is crucial to control. Diets that include fruits
and vegetables, especially those containing potassium, are helpful
for keeping blood pressure within normal ranges. Potassium has the
opposite effect of salt in the body—it lowers blood pressure naturally,
while salt raises it. Vegetables in the Under Pressure juice that are
high in potassium include tomato, bell pepper, carrots, and celery.
Vegetables and fruits that are natural diuretics are also crucial for
lowering blood pressure, such as cucumber, parsley, and lemon.*

2 LARGE CARROTS

1 MEDIUM GREEN BELL PEPPER

3 MEDIUM TOMATOES

3 LARGE CELERY STALKS

1 CUP PARSLEY

1 CUP CHOPPED SPINACH

½ ENGLISH CUCUMBER

Cut the ends off the carrots. Remove the stem from the bell pepper.
Juice the tomatoes, celery, carrots, and bell pepper. Push the parsley
and spinach through the juicer with the cucumber. Stir to combine
the juice before serving.

## INGREDIENTS TO LOWER HIGH BLOOD PRESSURE:

- Apple
- Asparagus
- Beet
- Bell pepper
- Blueberry
- Bok choy
- Broccoli
- Carrot
- Celery
- Cranberry
- Fig

- Garlic
- Grapes
- Kale
- Onion
- Orange
- Passion fruit
- Raspberry
- Spinach
- Strawberry
- Sweet potato
- Tomato

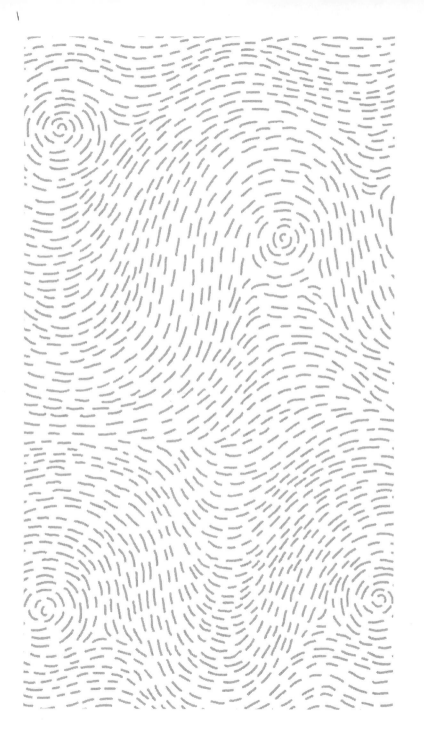

# CHAPTER SIX

# Immune System Support

CITRUS COUGH BUSTER

SUPERFOOD DETOX

FLU FIGHTER

FULL SYSTEM BOOST

GETTING A BOOST

KICK THE COLD

SAGE ADVICE FOR SORE THROAT

SPLENDID SINUSES

# Citrus Cough Buster

MAKES ABOUT 20 OUNCES, 3 SERVINGS

▶ CALORIES: 48, FAT: 0 G, SUGAR: 14 G, PROTEIN: 1 G,
CARBOHYDRATES: 15 G

*Foods high in vitamin C are natural immune boosters that can help your body fight both wet and dry coughs. The citrus fruit and cranberries in this rosy juice are packed with vitamin C. Vitamin A is also a powerful cough suppressant, and spinach is a wonderful source. You may add a spoonful of honey to the Citrus Cough Buster for a truly soothing remedy.*

2 LARGE ORANGES
1 GRAPEFRUIT
1 LIME
½ CUP CHOPPED SPINACH
½ CUP CRANBERRIES
PINCH OF CAYENNE PEPPER

Peel the oranges, grapefruit, and lime, leaving the pith, and cut them into quarters. Remove any visible seeds in the lime, because they will make the juice bitter. Juice the citrus fruit, alternating with the spinach and cranberries, until all the ingredients are used up. Stir the cayenne pepper into the juice before drinking.

**INGREDIENTS FOR COMBATING COUGHS:**

- Apple
- Apricot
- Asparagus
- Broccoli
- Cabbage
- Carrot
- Cayenne pepper
- Cranberry
- Grapefruit
- Green bell pepper
- Lemon
- Onion
- Orange
- Pear
- Pineapple
- Pumpkin
- Red bell pepper
- Spinach
- Turnip
- Watercress

# Superfood Detox

▶ CALORIES: 61, FAT: 0 G, SUGAR: 12 G, PROTEIN: 3 G, CARBOHYDRATES: 18 G

*This juice is simply good for every part of the body. It supports every system and organ. Apples are a superfood that support digestion and stabilize blood sugar. Beets detox the liver and support eye health. Carrots are packed with disease-fighting antioxidants and can boost immunity. Try this vibrant juice as a morning pick-me-up.*

2 MEDIUM GREEN APPLES
2 LARGE CARROTS
2 LEMONS
2 SMALL BEETS WITH GREENS
2 CUPS PARSLEY
1 SMALL ENGLISH CUCUMBER

Core and cut the apples into chunks. Cut the ends off the carrots. Peel the lemon, leaving the pith, and cut it in half. Remove any visible seeds. Juice the apples, beets, carrots, and lemons. Push the parsley through the juicer using the cucumber. Stir to combine the juice before drinking.

**INGREDIENTS FOR PROMOTING OVERALL GOOD HEALTH:**

- Apple
- Apricot
- Asparagus
- Beet
- Broccoli
- Brussels sprout
- Cantaloupe
- Carrot
- Corn
- Endive
- Fennel
- Fig
- Kale

- Kiwi
- Mango
- Nectarine
- Peach
- Pepper
- Pink grapefruit
- Pumpkin
- Radish
- Squash
- Spinach
- Sweet potato
- Tomatoes
- Watermelon

# Flu Fighter

MAKES ABOUT 12 OUNCES, 2 SERVINGS

▶ CALORIES: 49, FAT: 0 G, SUGAR: 8 G, PROTEIN: 2 G,
CARBOHYDRATES: 14 G

*The flu is a viral infection that causes more severe symptoms than the common cold. This juice is packed with antioxidants that can relieve these symptoms. Ginger is an antiviral that helps break up congestion and soothe a sore throat. Carrots help flush toxins from the body to eliminate fever and achy muscles. This juice is a good choice when you feel the flu first coming on.*

1 MEDIUM CARROT
1 SMALL GALA OR MACINTOSH APPLE
2 CUPS CHOPPED SPINACH
2 MEDIUM CELERY STALKS
ONE ½-INCH PIECE GINGER
½ SMALL ENGLISH CUCUMBER

Cut the end off the carrot. Core and chop the apple into chunks. Push the spinach through the juicer with the celery. Juice the carrot, apple, ginger, and cucumber. Stir to combine the juice before drinking.

**INGREDIENTS FOR FIGHTING THE FLU:**

- Apple
- Beet
- Broccoli
- Carrot
- Cayenne pepper
- Cranberry
- Fennel
- Garlic
- Ginger

- Grapefruit
- Kale
- Lemon
- Licorice
- Lime
- Orange
- Pineapple
- Radish

# Full System Boost

▶ CALORIES: 117, FAT: 1 G, SUGAR: 17 G, PROTEIN: 3 G, CARBOHYDRATES: 33 G

*Having a healthy, efficient immune system can make it possible for your body to fight off many illnesses, and it will also reduce your risk of developing chronic diseases such as heart disease and diabetes. Full System Boost juice uses the many antioxidants found in carrots, Swiss chard, and ginger to supercharge the immune system. Make this juice at least once a week during the cold and flu season to keep your body strong.*

2 LARGE CARROTS
2 GARLIC CLOVES
1 MEDIUM GREEN APPLE
ONE 1-INCH PIECE GINGER
1 CUP SWISS CHARD
1 CUP PARSLEY
PINCH OF GROUND CUMIN

Cut the ends off the carrots and peel the garlic cloves. Core the apple and cut it into quarters. Juice the carrots and ginger. Push the Swiss chard and parsley through the juicer using the apple wedges. Stir the cumin into the juice before drinking.

## INGREDIENTS FOR BOOSTING IMMUNITY:

- Apricot
- Asparagus
- Beet
- Broccoli
- Brussels sprout
- Butternut squash
- Cantaloupe
- Carrot
- Corn
- Honeydew melon
- Kale
- Kiwi

- Mango
- Nectarine
- Peach
- Pepper
- Pink grapefruit
- Pumpkin
- Spinach
- Squash
- Sweet potato
- Tomato
- Watermelon

# Getting a Boost

▶ CALORIES: 70, FAT: 1 G, SUGAR: 12 G, PROTEIN: 2 G,
CARBOHYDRATES: 20 G

*A healthy immune system is crucial to good overall health, and eating a broad range of fruits and vegetables in all different colors is key for getting immune-boosting antioxidants. The three main antioxidants in produce are beta-carotene and vitamins C and E. This juice is a nice mix of vegetables containing all three. Brussels sprouts, kiwi, and lemon are high in vitamin A, spinach is a good source of vitamin E, and carrots are packed with beta-carotene. The ginger is a powerful anti-inflammatory and tastes wonderful!*

4 KIWIS
3 MEDIUM CARROTS
1 LEMON
3 LARGE CELERY STALKS
1 BRUSSELS SPROUT
½ CUP CHOPPED SPINACH
ONE 1-INCH PIECE GINGER

Peel the kiwis and cut the ends off the carrots. Peel the lemon, leaving the pith, and cut it in half. Remove any visible seeds. Juice the celery, kiwi, carrots, Brussels sprout, spinach, and ginger. Juice the lemon last to wash out any ginger bits left in the juicer. Stir to combine the juice before drinking.

## INGREDIENTS FOR BOOSTING IMMUNITY:

- Apricot
- Asparagus
- Beet
- Broccoli
- Brussels sprout
- Butternut squash
- Cantaloupe
- Carrot
- Corn
- Honeydew melon
- Kale
- Kiwi

- Mango
- Nectarine
- Peach
- Pepper
- Pink grapefruit
- Pumpkin
- Spinach
- Squash
- Sweet potato
- Tomatoes
- Watermelon

# Kick the Cold

MAKES ABOUT 12 OUNCES, 1 SERVING

▶ CALORIES: 71, FAT: 1 G, SUGAR: 10 G, PROTEIN: 2 G,
   CARBOHYDRATES: 21 G

*Most people know that to fight a cold you need to eat citrus fruit. But did you know that another truly superior cold-fighting ingredient is garlic? This pungent addition to your juices has so many antibacterial properties that a cold won't stand a chance! Don't ignore citrus completely, because the lemon in this juice is an antiviral that can stop your cold from becoming truly nasty.*

1 PARSNIP
1 RED BELL PEPPER
1 GARLIC CLOVE
½ LEMON
4 RADISHES WITH GREENS
1 MEDIUM BEET WITH GREENS
½ SMALL ENGLISH CUCUMBER

Cut the end off the parsnip. Remove the stem from the red pepper. Peel the garlic clove. Peel the lemon, leaving the pith, and cut it in half. Remove any visible seeds. Juice the radishes, parsnip, beet, bell pepper, garlic, lemon, and cucumber. Stir to combine the juice before drinking.

## INGREDIENTS FOR FIGHTING THE COMMON COLD:

- Beet
- Carrot
- Cayenne pepper
- Cranberry
- Garlic
- Ginger
- Grapefruit
- Jicama
- Lemon
- Licorice
- Lime
- Orange
- Pineapple
- Radish

# Sage Advice for Sore Throat

MAKES ABOUT 12 OUNCES, 1 SERVING

▶ CALORIES: 110, FAT: 0 G, SUGAR: 23 G, PROTEIN: 2 G, CARBOHYDRATES: 31 G

*This delicious, soothing juice is designed to reduce the pain and scratchiness associated with a sore throat. The vitamin C in the orange and lemon is a traditional remedy for this type of health problem, and pineapple contains bromelain, which is also good for relieving sore throats. Sage is an antibacterial herb that can fight the actual source of the pain as well as reduce discomfort.*

1 LARGE ORANGE
½ LEMON
ONE 2-INCH SLICE PINEAPPLE
6 SAGE LEAVES
1 TABLESPOON HONEY

Peel the orange and lemon, leaving the pith, and cut the fruit in half. Remove the seeds from the lemon. Cut the pineapple into chunks. Juice the orange and pineapple. Juice the sage and lemon together. Stir the honey into the juice and drink immediately.

**INGREDIENTS TO FIGHT A SORE THROAT:**

- Banana
- Carrot
- Celery
- Cinnamon
- Ginger
- Green bell pepper
- Lemon
- Orange
- Pineapple
- Sage
- Spinach
- Tomato

# Splendid Sinuses

MAKES ABOUT 12 OUNCES, 1 SERVING

▶ CALORIES: 110, FAT: 1 G, SUGAR: 23 G, PROTEIN: 2 G,
CARBOHYDRATES: 35 G

*Ginger is a perfect ingredient to treat sinus problems, because the spicy-hot scent and taste of this powerful rhizome will tickle your nose and open up the sinus cavities. Vitamin C also supports a healthy respiratory tract, including the sinuses. Soon you will be breathing freely again, without pressure and congestion.*

1 GRANNY SMITH APPLE
1 LARGE ORANGE
1 LEMON
ONE 1½-INCH PIECE GINGER
PINCH OF CAYENNE PEPPER

Core and cut the apple into chunks. Peel the orange and lemon, leaving the pith, and cut them in half. Remove the seeds from the lemon. Juice the apple, orange, lemon, and ginger. Stir the cayenne pepper into the juice before drinking.

## INGREDIENTS FOR SINUSITIS AND SINUS PROBLEMS:

- Apple
- Beet
- Carrot
- Celery
- Cucumber
- Ginger
- Jalapeño pepper
- Lemon
- Lime
- Orange
- Parsley
- Radish
- Spinach
- Tomato

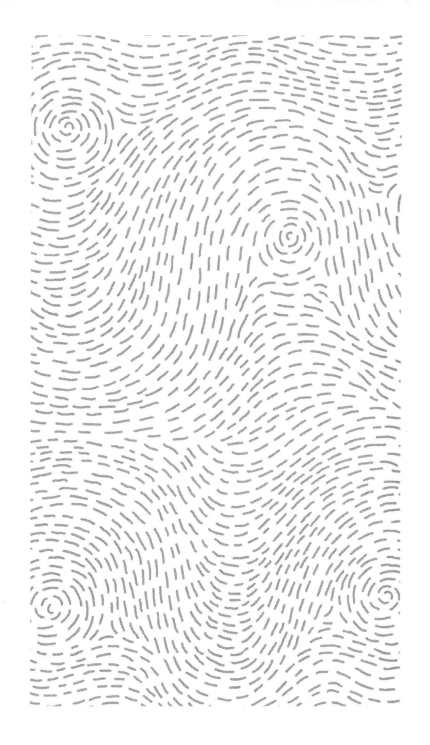

# CHAPTER SEVEN

# Weight Loss and Digestion Enhancers

ACID AWAY

BYE-BYE NAUSEA

DOES A BODY GOOD

EASY DIGESTION

GET THINGS MOVING

GOOD MORNING

GREEN HEARTBURN RELIEF

GUT FLORA BUILDER

IBS SUPPORT

MEAL IN A GLASS

METABOLISM MOVER

PAPAYA GUT REPRIEVE

# Acid Away

MAKES ABOUT 16 OUNCES, 2 SERVINGS

▶ CALORIES: 80, FAT: 1 G, SUGAR: 15 G, PROTEIN: 3 G,
CARBOHYDRATES: 25 G

*Gastroesophageal reflux disease (GERD) occurs when the contents of the stomach flow back upward, due to weak muscles between the stomach and esophagus. Eating the right foods and avoiding the wrong ones can heal and prevent this condition. Reducing the acidity in your stomach can be very beneficial, so that means eating soothing alkaline foods. The celery, cabbage, apples, and spinach in this juice are all alkaline. This combination can neutralize the acid in your stomach and heal or repair problems that cause GERD.*

2 GRANNY SMITH APPLES

3 LARGE CELERY STALKS

¼ HEAD WHITE CABBAGE

1 SMALL ENGLISH CUCUMBER

1 CUP CHOPPED SPINACH

½ CUP PARSLEY

ONE ½-INCH PIECE GINGER

Core the apples and cut them into chunks. Juice the celery, apples, and cabbage. Use the cucumber to push the spinach, parsley, and ginger through the juicer. Stir to combine the juice before drinking.

**INGREDIENTS FOR PREVENTING GERD:**

- Apple
- Avocado
- Banana
- Beet
- Broccoli
- Cabbage
- Carrot
- Celery
- Cucumber
- Fennel
- Jicama
- Kale
- Lemon
- Lemongrass
- Papaya
- Parsley
- Parsnip
- Spinach
- Watermelon

# Bye-Bye Nausea

MAKES ABOUT 20 OUNCES, 2 SERVINGS

▶ CALORIES: 122, FAT: 1 G, SUGAR: 19 G, PROTEIN: 6 G, CARBOHYDRATES: 37 G

*There are so many reasons why we might feel just plain nauseous. Often it is hard to pin down exactly what causes this stomach upset. However, Bye-Bye Nausea juice can offer you quick relief no matter what the reason (as long as it's not food poisoning—for which you really need to see a doctor). Apple gently cleanses, as does cucumber, which can also soothe stomach pain. Ginger is a centuries-old remedy for nausea, but don't add too much or the sweet taste of the carrots and apple will be masked.*

4 LARGE CARROTS
1 MEDIUM APPLE
1 PEAR
1 LEMON
ONE 1-INCH PIECE GINGER
1 CUP CHOPPED SPINACH
1 ENGLISH CUCUMBER

Cut the ends off the carrots. Core the apple and cut it into quarters, along with the pear. Peel the lemon, leaving the pith, and cut it in half. Remove any visible seeds. Juice the carrots, apple, pear, and ginger. Push the spinach through the juicer using the cucumber. Juice the lemon. Stir to combine the juices before drinking.

## INGREDIENTS TO RELIEVE NAUSEA:

- Apple
- Asparagus
- Beet
- Cabbage
- Carrot
- Celery
- Endive
- Fennel
- Fig
- Ginger
- Green bell pepper
- Kale
- Kiwi
- Lemon
- Orange
- Papaya
- Parsley
- Pear
- Romaine lettuce
- Spinach
- Strawberry
- Tomato
- Watermelon

# Does a Body Good

▶ CALORIES: 73, FAT: 1 G, SUGAR: 5 G, PROTEIN: 4 G, CARBOHYDRATES: 22 G

*You've lost weight, and now you want to maintain your body without rebounding back to previous scale numbers. Does a Body Good juice can be the perfect choice for a maintenance diet—it is filling and tastes great. Simply replace one meal with a serving of this juice, so your calorie intake stays within a healthful range. The orange and apple in this juice contain pectin, which is a natural appetite suppressant.*

1 LARGE GREEN APPLE
1 SMALL ORANGE
½ HEAD PURPLE CABBAGE
2 SMALL GREEN ZUCCHINI
1 CUP CAULIFLOWER FLORETS
1 CUP BLUEBERRIES
½ CUP KALE
½ SMALL ENGLISH CUCUMBER

Core the apple and cut it into wedges. Peel the orange, leaving the pith, and cut it into quarters. Cut the cabbage into chunks. Juice the zucchini, apple, cauliflower, and blueberries. Juice the orange and cabbage. Push the kale through the juicer using the cucumber. Stir to combine the juice before drinking.

**INGREDIENTS FOR WEIGHT MAINTENANCE:**

- Apple
- Asian pear
- Beet
- Brussels sprouts
- Cabbage
- Carrot
- Cauliflower
- Celery
- Collard greens
- Cucumber
- Jicama
- Kale
- Lemon
- Lime
- Orange
- Pear
- Spinach
- Tomato
- Zucchini

# Easy Digestion

MAKES ABOUT 16 OUNCES, 2 SERVINGS

▶  CALORIES: 65, FAT: 1 G, SUGAR: 10 G, PROTEIN: 2 G,
   CARBOHYDRATES: 20 G

*When your digestion is not in top working order, it may throw off your whole day. The best strategy is to fix the problem as quickly as possible with a tasty juice. Carrots are a sweet, satisfying base that also act as a cleanser to remove potential digestion irritants. Apples are so powerful and packed with nutrients that they should be consumed in some form every day. They also contain malic acid, which can improve digestion. This juice is rounded out by two proven digestive aids, fennel and ginger. Fennel can get things moving in your system, and the ginger can soothe an upset tummy while adding a little heat to this sweet juice.*

3 LARGE CARROTS
1 TART APPLE
2 LARGE CELERY STALKS
½ FENNEL BULB WITH GREENS
ONE 1-INCH PIECE GINGER

Cut the ends off the carrots. Core the apple and cut it into chunks. Juice the carrots, apple, celery, fennel, and ginger. Stir to combine the juice before drinking.

**INGREDIENTS TO AID DIGESTION:**

- Apple
- Asparagus
- Beet
- Cabbage
- Carrot
- Celery
- Endive
- Fennel
- Ginger
- Green bell pepper
- Kale
- Kiwi
- Lemon
- Orange
- Papaya
- Parsley
- Romaine lettuce
- Spinach
- Strawberry
- Tomato
- Watermelon

# Get Things Moving

▶ CALORIES: 137, FAT: 1 G, SUGAR: 24 G, PROTEIN: 4 G, CARBOHYDRATES: 42 G

*Fruits and vegetables are always a good choice when you are constipated, because fiber can keep you regular. Juicing produce removes the fiber, but the ingredients in juice are still an effective remedy to get you regular again. Apples are wonderful for getting things moving, but make sure you use a green apple—its enzymes are different. Spinach cleanses the digestive tract and keeps it healthy.*

8 LARGE CARROTS
2 KIWIS
½ LEMON
1 GREEN APPLE
1 LARGE BEET WITH GREENS
¼ CUP CHOPPED SPINACH

Cut the ends off the carrots. Peel the kiwis. Peel the lemon, leaving the pith, and cut it into wedges. Remove any visible seeds. Core the apple and cut into wedges. Juice the carrots, kiwis, apple, beet, spinach, and lemon. Stir to blend the juice before drinking.

**INGREDIENTS TO EASE CONSTIPATION AND PROMOTE REGULARITY:**

- Apple
- Asparagus
- Beet
- Cabbage
- Carrot
- Celery
- Fennel
- Ginger
- Green bell pepper
- Kale
- Kiwi
- Lemon
- Orange
- Papaya
- Parsley
- Pear
- Romaine lettuce
- Spinach
- Strawberry
- Tomato
- Watermelon

# Good Morning

MAKES ABOUT 16 OUNCES, 2 SERVINGS

▶ CALORIES: 92, FAT: 1 G, SUGAR: 17 G, PROTEIN: 2 G,
CARBOHYDRATES: 28 G

*Feeling nauseous and even vomiting are a very normal part of the first three months of pregnancy. Morning sickness can be awful, and what's worse is that it is not only in the morning! Fresh juiced vegetables and fruits can be a very effective way to get much-needed nutrients while lessoning the symptoms of morning sickness. Good Morning juice has a healthful helping of grapefruit, which can prevent diabetes in pregnancy and help settle the stomach. The apple and lemon in this juice also help support digestion.*

2 LARGE CARROTS
1 RUBY-RED GRAPEFRUIT
1 LEMON
1 APPLE
ONE 1-INCH PIECE GINGER

Cut the ends off the carrots. Peel the grapefruit and lemon, leaving the pith, and cut them into wedges. Remove the seeds from the lemon. Core the apple and cut it into wedges. Juice the carrot, grapefruit, apple, ginger, and lemon. Stir to combine the juice before drinking.

**INGREDIENTS TO EASE MORNING SICKNESS:**

- Apple
- Avocado
- Banana
- Cantaloupe
- Carrot
- Dragon fruit
- Grapefruit
- Lemon
- Lime
- Orange
- Papaya
- Spinach
- Strawberry
- Sweet potato
- Tomato
- Watercress

# Green Heartburn Relief

MAKES ABOUT 16 OUNCES, 2 SERVINGS

▶ CALORIES: 63, FAT: 1 G, SUGAR: 8 G, PROTEIN: 4 G,
CARBOHYDRATES: 12 G

*This juice is not really very green, but the broccoli and celery give it a greenish undertone. The combination of ingredients is very alkaline, which helps fight the acid of heartburn, and the sweet carrot helps this juice go down easy. Ginger is a natural remedy for digestion problems.*

4 LARGE CARROTS
2 LARGE CELERY STALKS
1 CUP BROCCOLI FLORETS
½ CUCUMBER
ONE 1-INCH PIECE GINGER
1 CUP CHOPPED COLLARD GREENS

Cut the ends off the carrots. Juice the carrots, celery, and broccoli. Use the cucumber to push the ginger and collard greens through the juicer. Stir to blend the juice before drinking.

## INGREDIENTS TO EASE HEARTBURN:

- Apple
- Avocado
- Banana
- Beet
- Broccoli
- Cabbage
- Carrot
- Celery
- Cucumber
- Jicama
- Kale
- Lemon
- Lemongrass
- Papaya
- Parsley
- Spinach
- Watermelon

# Gut Flora Builder

MAKES ABOUT 24 OUNCES, 3 SERVINGS

▶ CALORIES: 48, FAT: 0 G, SUGAR: 8 G, PROTEIN: 1 G, CARBOHYDRATES: 15 G

*You have trillions of bacteria living in your gut, some beneficial and some not. This bacteria is called gut flora, and it can help build a healthy immune system and fight disease if the good bacteria outnumber the bad. The apples in this juice can help decrease the bad bacteria and multiply the good. The garlic is a prebiotic that feeds the good bacteria and an antibiotic that reduces bad bacteria.*

2 GREEN APPLES
½ FENNEL WITH FRONDS
1 CARROT
½ LEMON
1 GARLIC CLOVE
2 LARGE CELERY STALKS

Core the apples and cut them into quarters. Cut the fennel into chunks. Cut the end off the carrot. Peel the lemon, leaving the pith, and cut it in half. Remove any visible seeds. Peel the skin off the garlic. Juice the apples, fennel, celery, carrot, garlic, and lemon. Stir to combine the juice before drinking.

## INGREDIENTS TO BUILD GOOD GUT FLORA:

- Apple
- Asparagus
- Beet
- Cabbage
- Carrot
- Celery
- Fennel
- Garlic
- Ginger
- Green bell pepper
- Kale
- Kiwi
- Lemon
- Orange
- Papaya
- Parsley
- Pear
- Romaine lettuce
- Spinach
- Strawberry
- Tomato
- Watermelon

# IBS Support

MAKES ABOUT 12 OUNCES, 1 SERVING

▶ CALORIES: 212, FAT: 2 G, SUGAR: 29 G, PROTEIN: 9 G, CARBOHYDRATES: 57 G

*Irritable bowel syndrome (IBS) is characterized by cramps, bloating, constipation, and diarrhea. It occurs when the food moving through the digestive tract travels too slow or too fast. Juicing is a wonderful way for people with IBS to get nutrients, because they often stick with white rice and white bread so that their symptoms don't flare up. Juices are very high in antioxidants, which can eliminate toxins in the body—especially helpful for slow transit problems. The apples in this fresh-tasting juice support a healthy digestive system, and ginger is very IBS-friendly.*

2 GREEN APPLES

¼ LEMON

6 KALE LEAVES

½ CUP PARSLEY

¼ CUP CILANTRO

ONE 1-INCH PIECE GINGER

2 LARGE CELERY STALKS

Core the apples and chop them into chunks. Peel the lemon, leaving the pith, and cut it in half. Remove any visible seeds. Juice the apple. Push the kale, parsley, cilantro, and ginger through the juicer using the celery. Juice the lemon. Stir to combine the juice before serving.

## INGREDIENTS TO EASE IBS:

- Apple
- Banana
- Bell pepper
- Blueberry
- Bok choy
- Carrots
- Celery
- Cilantro
- Eggplant
- Endive
- Fennel
- Grape

- Grapefruit
- Green bean
- Honeydew
- Kale
- Kiwi
- Lemon
- Lettuce
- Lime
- Parsnip
- Pumpkin
- Sweet potato
- Tomato

# Meal in a Glass

▶ CALORIES: 72, FAT: 1 G, SUGAR: 13 G, PROTEIN: 3 G,
CARBOHYDRATES: 25 G

*Losing weight is really just simple math. You need to consume fewer calories than you burn. Juicing can be a good way to accelerate weight loss, as long as you remember that juice may actually have a fair number of calories if the juice is predominantly fruit. Pretty much any combination of vegetables (and one or two fruits in moderation) can create a low-calorie, fat-free, antioxidant-packed treat that is just the thing when you need a boost.*

4 MEDIUM CARROTS
½ LEMON
1 RED DELICIOUS APPLE
4 BRUSSELS SPROUTS
2 MEDIUM TOMATOES
1 ASIAN PEAR
1 MEDIUM BEET WITH GREENS
½ CUP WHITE CAULIFLOWER FLORETS
½ CUP BROCCOLI FLORETS

Cut the ends off the carrots. Peel the lemon, leaving the pith, and cut it in half. Remove any visible seeds. Core the apple and cut it into chunks. Juice the Brussels sprouts, carrots, apple, tomatoes, pear, beet, cauliflower, broccoli, and lemon. Stir to combine the juice before drinking.

## INGREDIENTS TO PROMOTE WEIGHT LOSS:

- Apple
- Asian pear
- Beet
- Brussels sprout
- Carrot
- Cauliflower
- Celery
- Collard greens
- Cucumber
- Jicama
- Kale
- Lemon
- Lime
- Orange
- Pear
- Spinach
- Tomato

# Metabolism Mover

MAKES ABOUT 16 OUNCES, 2 SERVINGS

▶  CALORIES: 94, FAT: 1 G, SUGAR: 19 G, PROTEIN: 3 G,
   CARBOHYDRATES: 27 G

*Metabolism is how fast or slow your body converts the food you eat
into energy. Metabolism depends on age, body type, exercise level,
gender, and other factors that are not entirely understood. Having a
slow metabolism can make you susceptible to weight gain. Studies
have shown that the resting metabolism of older adults can be boosted
when oxidative stress is removed using produce rich in vitamin C, like
lemons. The grapefruit in this juice also increases metabolism and
stabilizes insulin levels. This juice should be consumed in the morning
to start your day off right.*

1 GREEN APPLE
1 RUBY-RED GRAPEFRUIT
½ LEMON
1 SMALL ENGLISH CUCUMBER
1 BEET WITH GREENS
ONE ½-INCH PIECE GINGER

Core the apple and chop it into chunks. Peel the grapefruit and
lemon, leaving the pith, and cut them into quarters. Remove the
seeds from the lemon. Juice the apple, cucumber, beet, grapefruit,
lemon, and ginger. Stir to blend the juice before drinking.

**INGREDIENTS FOR BOOSTING METABOLISM:**

- Apple
- Blueberry
- Broccoli
- Carrot
- Celery
- Grape
- Grapefruit
- Green bean
- Green bell pepper
- Melon
- Orange
- Parsley
- Radish
- Red bell pepper
- Spinach
- Spring onion
- Strawberry
- Tomato

# Papaya Gut Reprieve

MAKES ABOUT 12 OUNCES, 1 SERVING

▶ CALORIES: 149, FAT: 2 G, SUGAR: 13 G, PROTEIN: 9 G,
CARBOHYDRATES: 37 G

*It should be no surprise that you can improve your digestion and get rid of uncomfortable gas with food, because food causes digestive problems in the first place. This pretty juice is flavored simply with ginger and lemon to soothe a tender gut and relax the intestinal tract, which reduces gas. The cabbage provides the bulk of the juice and clears out whatever might be causing the gas in the stomach. The papaya adds color and a sweet taste along with papain to speed protein digestion.*

1 SMALL PAPAYA
½ LEMON
6 KALE LEAVES
¼ HEAD CABBAGE
ONE 1½-INCH PIECE GINGER

Peel and seed the papaya. Peel the lemon, leaving the pith, and cut it in half. Remove any visible seeds. Juice the kale, papaya, and cabbage, using the chunks of fruit to push the kale through the juicer. Juice the ginger and lemon. Stir to combine the juice before drinking.

**INGREDIENTS TO SOOTHE GAS AND BLOATING:**

- Apple
- Asparagus
- Beet
- Cabbage
- Carrot
- Celery
- Endive
- Fennel
- Ginger
- Green bell pepper
- Kale
- Kiwi
- Lemon
- Orange
- Papaya
- Parsley
- Romaine lettuce
- Spinach
- Strawberry
- Tomato
- Watermelon

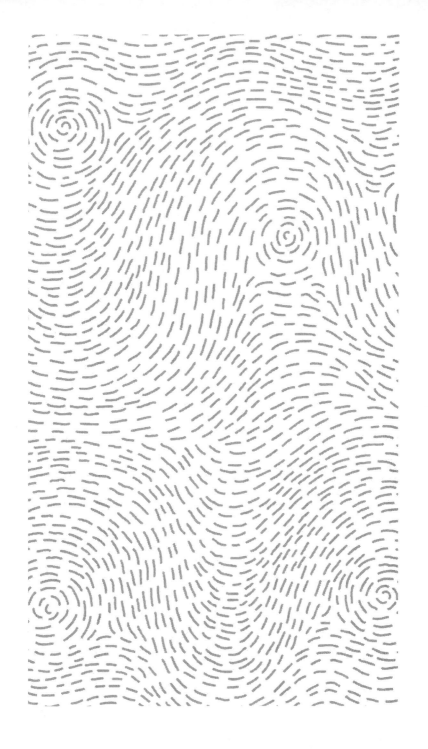

# CHAPTER EIGHT

# Cancer and Disease Prevention

BETTER BODY

BONNY BONE
FRUIT SURPRISE

CUTTING CANCER

GOUT BE GONE

HAPPY COLON

HEALTHFUL HEART
GINGER

PROMOTE PROSTATE
HEALTH

BEAT BREAST CANCER

THYROID BUDDY

# Better Body

MAKES ABOUT 20 OUNCES, 2 SERVINGS

▶ CALORIES: 29, FAT: 1 G, SUGAR: 9 G, PROTEIN: 3 G, CARBOHYDRATES: 21 G

*Leukemia is a cancer that starts in the bone marrow and spreads to the blood. As with other cancers, good nutrition can help in treatment, and juicing is an effective way to get the nutrients that are important. Studies have shown that carrots help in the fight against leukemia, and they figure prominently in this vibrant-hued juice. Beets contain potent cancer-fighting compounds, too, such as betacyanins, which also give beets their glorious color.*

3 LARGE CARROTS

1 LIME

1 JALAPEÑO PEPPER

1 LARGE BEET WITH GREENS

2 CUPS CHOPPED SPINACH

2 LARGE CELERY STALKS

ONE 1-INCH PIECE GINGER

Cut the ends off the carrots. Peel the lime, leaving the pith, and cut the fruit into quarters. Remove any seeds. Cut the jalapeño pepper in half, and remove the seeds, if desired, for less heat. Juice the carrots and beet. Push the spinach through the juicer using the celery stalks. Juice the ginger, jalapeño pepper, and lime. Stir to combine the juice before drinking.

**INGREDIENTS TO HELP FIGHT LEUKEMIA:**

- Beet
- Carrot
- Cayenne pepper
- Celeriac
- Celery
- Collard greens
- Cucumber
- Dandelion

- Garlic
- Ginger
- Kale
- Parsley
- Pepper
- Radish
- Spinach
- Wheatgrass

# Bonny Bone Fruit Surprise

MAKES ABOUT 16 OUNCES, 2 SERVINGS

▶ CALORIES: 95, FAT: 1 G, SUGAR: 18 G, PROTEIN: 2 G, CARBOHYDRATES: 31 G

*Osteoporosis literally means "porous bone," and that is what this disease does. It can cause fractures and a characteristic hunched-over spine. A diet rich in fruits and vegetables can be instrumental in preventing this devastating disease; in particular, the most useful fruits and vegetables are those rich in calcium and vitamins C and D. Calcium is the building block of bone, but it is only absorbed into the bones in the presence of vitamin D. Studies have shown that vitamin C, which creates an acidic environment in the body, can also promote better calcium uptake.*

1 KIWI
1 MEDIUM PEAR
1 CUP BLACKBERRIES
¼ PINEAPPLE
1 CUP MINT LEAVES

Peel the kiwi. Cut the pear into quarters. Juice the kiwi, blackberries, and pear together. Cut the pineapple into chunks. Juice the mint and pineapple together, using the pineapple to push the leaves through. Stir to combine the juice before drinking.

**INGREDIENTS TO PREVENT OSTEOPOROSIS:**

- Apple
- Asparagus
- Blackberry
- Bok choy
- Broccoli
- Brussels sprout
- Cabbage
- Carrot
- Cherry
- Citrus fruit
- Cranberry
- Endive
- Fig
- Grape
- Jicama
- Kiwi
- Parsnip
- Pear
- Pineapple
- Radish
- Spinach
- Turnip

# Cutting Cancer

MAKES ABOUT 16 OUNCES, 2 SERVINGS

▶ CALORIES: 84, FAT: 1 G, SUGAR: 10 G, PROTEIN: 4 G,
CARBOHYDRATES: 21 G

*There are few diseases that strike more fear than cancer. Studies have shown that food choices can be very important when it comes to preventing cancer. Fruits and vegetables in their natural form are the healthiest, and juicing provides all the goodness of the produce. This cancer-preventing juice is very rich in beta-carotene, which can slow the multiplication of cancer cells. Kale is high in flavonoids and carotenoids, which have many more anticancer benefits.*

2 LARGE CARROTS
1 GRANNY SMITH APPLE
1 MEDIUM ORANGE BELL PEPPER
1 CUP CHOPPED COLLARD GREENS
½ CUP CILANTRO
½ CUP CHOPPED KALE

Cut the ends off the carrots. Core the apple and cut it into wedges. Take the stem out of the bell pepper and cut it into quarters. Juice the carrots and apple. Push the collard greens, cilantro, and kale through the juicer using the bell pepper. Stir to combine the juice before drinking.

## INGREDIENTS TO HELP PREVENT CANCER:

- Apple
- Apricot
- Asparagus
- Banana
- Bok choy
- Broccoli
- Cantaloupe
- Cilantro
- Collard greens
- Ginger
- Honeydew melon
- Kale
- Kiwi
- Lemon
- Mango
- Nectarine
- Orange
- Pear
- Pepper
- Spinach
- Strawberry
- Swiss chard
- Tomato
- Turmeric
- Watermelon

# Gout Be Gone

MAKES ABOUT 24 OUNCES, 3 SERVINGS

▶ CALORIES: 53, FAT: 0 G, SUGAR: 10 G, PROTEIN: 1 G, CARBOHYDRATES: 16 G

*Gout is a painful condition caused by excessive amounts of uric acid in the body. This causes the blood to be highly acidic and creates pain in the extremities as the uric acid crystallizes, particularly in the feet. The main ingredient in this dark juice is cherries, which can lower the amount of uric acid in the body. Make sure you drink at least eight glasses of water a day along with juices like this one to lower your risk of gout.*

1 CUP BLACK CHERRIES
1 GRANNY SMITH APPLE
1 LARGE CARROT
¼ LEMON
2 LARGE CELERY STALKS
½ SMALL ENGLISH CUCUMBER

Pit the cherries. Core the apple and cut it into wedges. Cut the end off the carrot. Peel the lemon, leaving the pith, and cut it in half. Remove any visible seeds. Juice the cherries, apple, carrot, celery, cucumber, and lemon. Stir to combine the juice before drinking.

## INGREDIENTS TO PREVENT AND EASE GOUT:

- Asparagus
- Beet
- Blueberry
- Carrot
- Celery
- Cherry
- Cucumber

- Green apple
- Guava
- Lemon
- Lemongrass
- Lime
- Orange

# Happy Colon

▶ CALORIES: 80, FAT: 0 G, SUGAR: 13 G, PROTEIN: 2 G, CARBOHYDRATES: 26 G

*Nutrition is a powerful weapon in preventing colon cancer. The general advice is to reduce the saturated fat in your diet and include an array of colorful vegetables and fruits that are rich in nutrients and antioxidants. Cranberries have potent anticancer properties. The oranges, grapefruit, and limes in this juice contain bioflavonoids and vitamin C, which may reduce the risk of colon cancer.*

2 ORANGES
1 LARGE GRAPEFRUIT
2 LIMES
3 CUPS CRANBERRIES
ONE 2-INCH PIECE GINGER
HONEY TO SWEETEN, IF NEEDED

Peel the oranges, grapefruit, and limes, leaving the pith. Cut the fruit into quarters. Remove the seeds from the lime. Juice the cranberries, alternating with the citrus fruits and ginger, until everything is used up. Stir to combine the juice and sweeten it with honey, if using, before drinking.

## INGREDIENTS TO PREVENT COLON CANCER:

- Apple
- Brussels sprout
- Cauliflower
- Celery
- Cranberry
- Cucumber
- Ginger
- Grapefruit
- Green bell pepper
- Lemon
- Lime
- Orange
- Peach
- Pineapple
- Radish
- Spinach
- Sweet potato
- Tomato
- Watermelon

# Healthful Heart Ginger

MAKES ABOUT 16 OUNCES, 2 SERVINGS

▶ CALORIES: 95, FAT: 1 G, SUGAR: 16 G, PROTEIN: 3 G, CARBOHYDRATES: 29 G

*Heart disease is the number one killer of both men and women in the United States, so prevention should be on the top of every healthful lifestyle list. Healthful Heart Ginger juice is a wonderful all-around cardiovascular system tonic that combats high cholesterol, atherosclerosis, and high blood pressure. There are many nutrients that are important to heart health, such as magnesium, in spinach and other dark, leafy greens. Potassium, another key nutrient, is found in cucumber. Vitamin C is an antioxidant found in apples, cucumber, and papaya.*

1 GREEN APPLE

1 PEAR

½ PAPAYA

2 LARGE CELERY STALKS

2 CUPS CHOPPED SPINACH

1 CUP PARSLEY

ONE 2-INCH PIECE GINGER

1 SMALL ENGLISH CUCUMBER

Core the apple and cut it into wedges. Cut the pear into quarters. Peel the papaya and scoop out the seeds, because they may make the juice bitter. Juice the celery, apple, and pear. Juice the spinach, parsley, ginger, and papaya, pushing it through the juicer with the cucumber. Stir to combine the juice before drinking.

## INGREDIENTS TO PREVENT HEART DISEASE:

- Apple
- Blackberry
- Blueberry
- Broccoli
- Carrot
- Collard greens
- Cucumber
- Garlic
- Kale
- Kiwi
- Orange
- Papaya
- Parsley
- Parsnip
- Passion fruit
- Raspberry
- Red grape
- Spinach
- Strawberry
- Tomato
- Watermelon

# Promote Prostate Health

MAKES ABOUT 16 OUNCES, 2 SERVINGS

▶ CALORIES: 134, FAT: 0 G, SUGAR: 27 G, PROTEIN: 3 G,
CARBOHYDRATES: 38 G

*In the United States, prostate cancer is the most common cancer in men. Nutrition in general, and specifically juicing, can help reduce the risk of developing this cancer. This sweet juice is mostly watermelon, which is high in lycopene, a nutrient that has been shown in studies to reduce the risk of prostate cancer. Blueberries are another delicious ingredient in this juice, and they have been found to block the development, promotion, and spread of prostate cancer cells.*

1 LIME
6 CUPS DICED WATERMELON
¼ CUP BASIL
1½ CUPS BLUEBERRIES
PINCH OF CAYENNE PEPPER

Cut the peel off the lime, leaving the pith, and cut it into quarters. Remove any seeds. Peel the outer skin off the watermelon, leaving as much rind as possible. Juice the basil, blueberries, and lime. Juice the watermelon. Stir the cayenne pepper into the juice before drinking.

**INGREDIENTS TO PREVENT PROSTATE CANCER:**

- Apple
- Apricot
- Blueberry
- Broccoli
- Brussels sprout
- Cabbage
- Cantaloupe
- Carrot
- Celery
- Garlic
- Grapefruit
- Kale
- Lemon
- Papaya
- Pear
- Pomegranate
- Red bell pepper
- Spinach
- Tomato
- Watermelon

# Beat Breast Cancer

MAKES ABOUT 16 OUNCES, 2 SERVINGS

▶ CALORIES: 64, FAT: 1 G, SUGAR: 8 G, PROTEIN: 4 G, CARBOHYDRATES: 19 G

*Breast cancer is thought to develop in one out of eight women younger than eighty-five. Fruits and vegetables are powerful medicines against this all-too-common disease, and Beat Breast Cancer juice has several potent ingredients that may help prevent it. Parsley and celery contain a compound called apigenin, which can prevent certain types of breast cancer cells from growing. Turmeric has an active ingredient called curcumin that has been linked to preventing breast cancer metastasis.*

½ LEMON

2 KIWIS

4 LARGE CELERY STALKS

½ CUP PARSLEY

1 CUP CHOPPED SWISS CHARD

½ SMALL ENGLISH CUCUMBER

1 CUP BROCCOLI FLORETS

ONE 1-INCH PIECE GINGER

PINCH OF TURMERIC

Peel the lemon, leaving the pith, and cut it into wedges. Remove any seeds. Peel and juice the kiwis. Juice the celery, parsley, and Swiss chard, using the cucumber to push the leaves through. Juice the broccoli, ginger, and lemon. Stir the turmeric into the juice before drinking.

**INGREDIENTS TO FIGHT BREAST CANCER:**

- Apple
- Asparagus
- Broccoli
- Cilantro
- Collard greens
- Ginger
- Kale
- Kiwi
- Lemon
- Orange
- Pear
- Pepper
- Spinach
- Strawberry
- Swiss chard
- Tomato
- Turmeric
- Watermelon

# Thyroid Buddy

MAKES ABOUT 16 OUNCES, 2 SERVINGS

▶ CALORIES: 111, FAT: 1 G, SUGAR: 22 G, PROTEIN: 4 G,
CARBOHYDRATES: 35 G

*The thyroid is a very small gland with a very big job. It releases hormones required to regulate many body functions, including metabolism, growth, and maturation. If it does not release enough hormones, weight gain, depression, increased cholesterol, and fatigue may result. These are symptoms of hypothyroidism (underactive thyroid). This tart juice contains two ingredients that are high in iodine, which is required to keep the thyroid functioning properly: watercress and cranberries.*

2 RED DELICIOUS APPLES
½ LEMON
1 POUND WATERCRESS
¼ FENNEL WITH FRONDS
¼ CUP CRANBERRIES

Core the apples and cut them into wedges. Peel the lemon, leaving the pith, and cut it into wedges. Remove any seeds. Juice the watercress, using the apples and fennel to push it through the juicer. Juice the cranberries and lemon. Stir to combine the juice before serving.

## INGREDIENTS TO PREVENT AND MANAGE HYPOTHYROIDISM:

- Apple
- Apricot
- Avocado
- Banana
- Beet
- Bell pepper
- Blackberry
- Blueberry
- Carrot
- Celery
- Cherry
- Cranberry
- Cucumber
- Papaya
- Pepper
- Pineapple
- Pumpkin
- Squash
- Tomato
- Zucchini

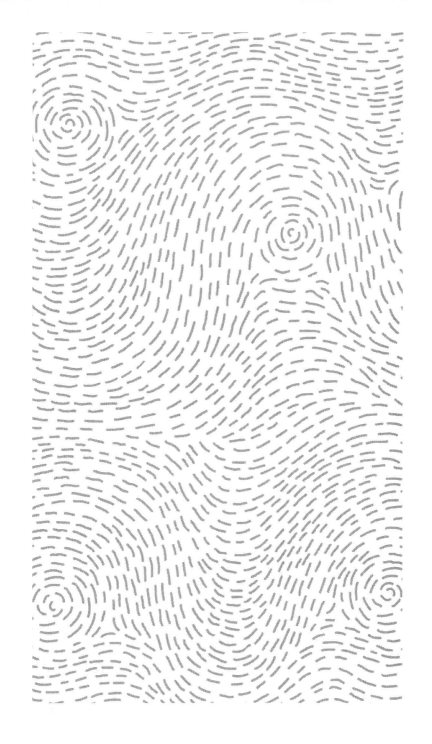

# CHAPTER NINE

# Energy and Vitality Boost

AFTERMATH RECOVERY

BEFORE GYM BLITZ

BURN, BABY, BURN

FAT FURNACE

GREEN GO-GO

PICK ME UP

READY TO RECOVER

SLOW ENERGY

# Aftermath Recovery

MAKES ABOUT 20 OUNCES, 2 SERVINGS

▶ CALORIES: 133, FAT: 2 G, SUGAR: 10 G, PROTEIN: 14 G, CARBOHYDRATES: 36 G

*The effects of a good workout do not end when you step off the equipment or put down the weights at the end of your last set. Your body continues to burn fat and glucose for hours afterward. Feed this need with a recovery juice. Spinach is crucial for building strength because it contains compounds called phytoecdysteroids, which can increase muscle growth. The lemon in this tart, slightly bitter juice helps ramp up the metabolism so you burn more fat post-workout. If this juice is too earthy and bitter for your taste, add a green apple to mellow it out.*

1 LEMON

1 CUP CHOPPED SPINACH

2 LARGE KALE LEAVES

½ CUP BROCCOLI FLORETS

1 CUCUMBER

½ CUP BLACKBERRIES

Peel the lemon, leaving the pith, and cut it in half. Remove any seeds. Juice the spinach, kale, and broccoli, using the broccoli to press the spinach through the juicer. Juice the cucumber, blackberries, and lemon. Stir to combine the juices before drinking.

**INGREDIENTS FOR BETTER POST-WORKOUT RECOVERY:**

- Asparagus
- Avocado
- Beet
- Bell pepper
- Blackberry
- Blueberry
- Broccoli
- Cabbage
- Carrot
- Celery
- Cilantro
- Cucumber

- Grapefruit
- Hot pepper
- Kale
- Lime
- Mango
- Parsley
- Pear
- Raspberry
- Spinach
- Strawberry
- Sweet potato
- Watermelon

# Before Gym Blitz

MAKES ABOUT 28 OUNCES, 3 SERVINGS

▶ CALORIES: 66, FAT: 1 G, SUGAR: 11 G, PROTEIN: 4 G,
CARBOHYDRATES: 21 G

*This very green juice should be consumed about half an hour before you work out or engage in physical activity. Spinach makes this juice so green; it's high in calcium, which prevents muscle cramping and allows for better muscle contractions, meaning you'll get more from your workouts. If your workouts are geared toward weight loss as well, the cilantro will help you reach that goal. It triggers waste removal from the body and supports a healthy digestive system, which are key to weight loss.*

2 GRANNY SMITH APPLES
½ LEMON
1 BUNCH SPINACH
1 CUP CILANTRO
1 HEAD ROMAINE LETTUCE
6 TO 7 MINT LEAVES

Core and cut the apples into quarters. Peel the lemon, leaving the pith, and cut it into wedges. Remove any seeds. Juice the spinach, cilantro, and apples, using the apples to push the spinach and cilantro through the juicer. Juice the romaine, lemon, and mint. Stir to combine the juice before drinking.

## INGREDIENTS FOR BEFORE A WORKOUT:

- Apple
- Asparagus
- Beet
- Bell pepper
- Blackberry
- Blueberry
- Cabbage
- Carrot
- Celery
- Cilantro

- Cucumber
- Grapefruit
- Hot pepper
- Mango
- Pear
- Raspberry
- Spinach
- Strawberry
- Sweet potato
- Watermelon

# Burn, Baby, Burn

MAKES ABOUT 20 OUNCES, 3 SERVINGS

▶ CALORIES: 110, FAT: 1 G, SUGAR: 17 G, PROTEIN: 3 G, CARBOHYDRATES: 31 G

*This juice is good for stoking up the metabolic fire in the body. It is a sunny yellow color that guarantees a smile. Pineapple provides sweetness and also contains an enzyme that boosts the metabolism and can accelerate weight loss. One small kiwi has about twice the recommended daily amount of vitamin C, an essential nutrient linked to a higher-revving metabolism.*

½ SMALL PINEAPPLE
3 LARGE KIWIS
1 LARGE YELLOW BELL PEPPER
1 CUP SWEET CORN
½ ENGLISH CUCUMBER

Cut the pineapple into chunks, leaving the skin and core. If your juicer instructions indicate that the machine cannot handle these parts of the fruit, peel and core the pineapple. Peel the kiwis. Take the stem out of the bell pepper and cut it in half. Juice the pineapple, kiwis, bell pepper, corn, and cucumber. Stir to combine the juices before drinking.

**INGREDIENTS TO BOOST METABOLISM:**

- Asparagus
- Avocado
- Bell pepper
- Cinnamon
- Honeydew melon
- Hot pepper
- Kiwi
- Mango
- Pineapple
- Spinach
- Tomato
- Watermelon

# Fat Furnace

MAKES ABOUT 24 OUNCES, 3 SERVINGS

▶ CALORIES: 48, FAT: 0 G, SUGAR: 10 G, PROTEIN: 1 G, CARBOHYDRATES: 14 G

*Many people begin juicing with the idea that they will lose a great deal of weight. This may be true for a juice cleanse, but that's only for a few days. And simply including more juices in your diet will not make you lose weight. The healthiest way to use juice is to simply help your body burn a little more fat. In this sunny juice, you'll combine grapefruit—which contains enzymes that lower insulin levels, thus cutting cravings and preventing fat storage—with carrots. Carrots are very high in beta-carotene, which flushes fat out of your system.*

1 RUBY-RED GRAPEFRUIT
1 ORANGE
2 SMALL CARROTS
2 LARGE CELERY STALKS
2 RADISHES WITH GREENS
ONE ½-INCH PIECE GINGER
PINCH OF CAYENNE PEPPER

Peel the grapefruit and orange, leaving the pith, and cut them into quarters. Cut the ends off the carrots. Juice the grapefruit, orange, carrots, celery, radishes, and ginger. Stir the cayenne pepper into the juice before drinking.

## INGREDIENTS TO BURN FAT:

- Apple
- Asparagus
- Beet
- Bell pepper
- Blackberry
- Blueberry
- Cabbage
- Carrot
- Celery
- Cucumber
- Grapefruit
- Hot pepper
- Mango
- Pear
- Raspberry
- Strawberry
- Sweet potato
- Watermelon

# Green Go-Go

▶ CALORIES: 62, FAT: 1 G, SUGAR: 4 G, PROTEIN: 5 G,
CARBOHYDRATES: 15 G

*Flagging energy during a workout may hamper motivation. There are some wonderful juices you can drink while on the go or working out that will ensure you have enough energy to finish strong. Parsley is high in protein, which is crucial for building and nourishing strong muscles. Cucumbers are often thought of as the hydrating vegetable in fresh juices. They are also a wonderful source of silicon, which can improve flexibility and mobility by improving the elasticity of the joints.*

½ LIME
1 PEAR
1 CUP PARSLEY
1 CUP CHOPPED KALE
½ CUP CHOPPED SPINACH
2 LARGE CELERY STALKS
½ SMALL ENGLISH CUCUMBER

Peel the lime, leaving the pith, and cut it into wedges. Remove any seeds. Cut the pear in half. Juice the parsley, kale, and spinach, pushing it through with the celery. Juice the cucumber, pear, and lime. Stir to combine the juice before serving.

## INGREDIENTS FOR WORKOUT STAMINA:

- Apple
- Asparagus
- Beet
- Bell pepper
- Blackberry
- Blueberry
- Cabbage
- Carrot
- Celery
- Cilantro
- Cucumber
- Grapefruit
- Hot pepper
- Kale
- Lime
- Mango
- Parsley
- Pear
- Raspberry
- Spinach
- Strawberry
- Sweet potato
- Watermelon

# Pick Me Up

MAKES ABOUT 24 OUNCES, 3 SERVINGS

▶ CALORIES: 121, FAT: 1 G, SUGAR: 21 G, PROTEIN: 4 G,
CARBOHYDRATES: 36 G

*If you have ever ended up crashing from fatigue in the midafternoon, you will appreciate what a quick drink of fresh juice can do for your flagging energy. Pumpkin might seem like an odd juicing choice, but it is sweet and provides sustained energy to combat fatigue. Polyphenol from apples has been linked in several studies to reducing fatigue, so it is a very good addition to this juice—and it adds a nice touch of sweetness.*

1 MEDIUM PUMPKIN
1 GRANNY SMITH APPLE
2 LARGE CARROTS
3 LARGE CELERY STALKS
2 CUPS CHOPPED SPINACH
½ ENGLISH CUCUMBER

Peel and seed the pumpkin, and cut it into small chunks. Core the apple and cut it into wedges. Cut the ends off the carrots. Juice the pumpkin, apple, carrots, and celery. Juice the spinach, pushing it through with the cucumber. Stir to combine the juice before drinking.

**INGREDIENTS TO COMBAT FATIGUE:**

- Apple
- Asparagus
- Beet
- Bell pepper
- Blackberry
- Blueberry
- Cabbage
- Carrot
- Celery
- Cilantro
- Cucumber
- Grapefruit

- Hot pepper
- Kale
- Lime
- Mango
- Parsley
- Pear
- Pumpkin
- Raspberry
- Spinach
- Strawberry
- Sweet potato
- Watermelon

# Ready to Recover

MAKES ABOUT 24 OUNCES, 3 SERVINGS

▶ CALORIES: 106, FAT: 4 G, SUGAR: 15 G, PROTEIN: 3 G,
CARBOHYDRATES: 24 G

*Exercise experts agree that you need to let your body rest between workouts. You can stall your weight loss or muscle gain plans by overtraining. One important aspect of resting your body is feeding it the nutrients it needs to recover. To help your body recover, this juice should be whipped up about four hours after you are done exercising. Carotenoid-rich avocado is important for boosting your immune system after working out, because your immunity is lower after exercising. Broccoli is high in chromium, which helps the body metabolize protein to be used by your tired muscles.*

1 GRANNY SMITH APPLE

2 SMALL ORANGES

1 SMALL BANANA

½ UNDER-RIPE AVOCADO

10 CHERRIES, PITTED

1 BROCCOLI STALK

½ TEASPOON GROUND CINNAMON

Core and cut the apple into wedges. Peel the oranges, leaving the pith, and cut them into quarters. Peel the banana. Peel the avocado and remove the pit. Juice the apple, cherries, banana, and broccoli. Juice 1 orange, using it to push the previous ingredients through. Juice the avocado with the remaining orange. Stir the cinnamon into the juice before drinking.

## INGREDIENTS FOR MUSCLE RECOVERY:

- Asparagus
- Avocado
- Banana
- Beet
- Bell pepper
- Blackberry
- Blueberry
- Broccoli
- Cabbage
- Carrot
- Celery
- Cherry
- Cucumber
- Grapefruit
- Kale
- Lime
- Mango
- Parsley
- Pear
- Raspberry
- Spinach
- Strawberry
- Sweet potato
- Watermelon

# Slow Energy

MAKES ABOUT 16 OUNCES, 2 SERVINGS

▶ CALORIES: 76, FAT: 1 G, SUGAR: 15 G, PROTEIN: 2 G,
CARBOHYDRATES: 24 G

*Juices can be quite high in calories and sugar if there is a lot of fruit in them or if the produce is high on the glycemic index (GI). The GI measures how much carbohydrates from food raise your blood sugar after eating them. It's a ranking from zero to one hundred; foods with a GI value of 55 or below are considered healthier. This juice uses only low-GI foods, so it is a very good choice for people with diabetes, or for those times when you need slow, sustained energy to get through the day.*

½ LEMON
2 GRANNY SMITH APPLES
4 CELERY STALKS
ONE 1-INCH PIECE GINGER
1 CUP PARSLEY

Peel the lemon, leaving the pith, and quarter it. Remove any seeds. Core the apples and cut them into chunks. Juice the apples. Juice the celery, ginger, parsley, and lemon. Stir to combine the juice before drinking.

## INGREDIENTS FOR LOW GLYCEMIC INDEX JUICES:

- Apple
- Broccoli
- Cabbage
- Carrot
- Cauliflower
- Celery
- Cherry
- Cucumber
- Grapefruit
- Green bean
- Hot pepper
- Kiwi
- Lettuce
- Onion
- Orange
- Peach
- Pear
- Plum
- Red bell pepper
- Strawberry
- Tomato

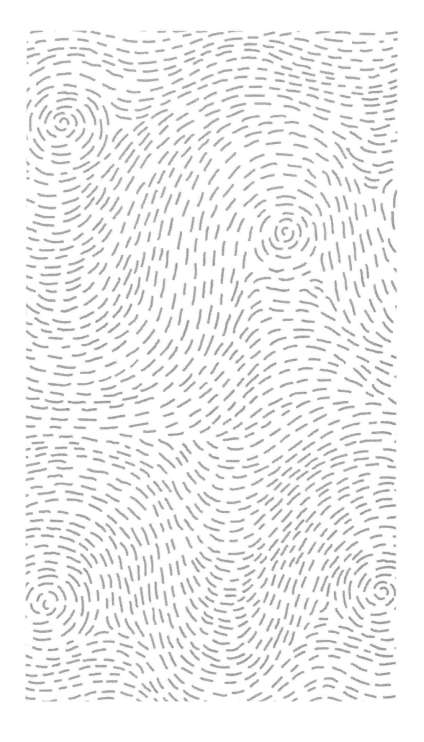

# CHAPTER TEN

# Taming Inflammation

ALLERGY RELIEF

ASPARAGUS ARTHRITIS
RELIEF

BREATHE EASY

GLOWING GINSENG

INFLAMMATION BUSTER

LIQUID CHLOROPHYLL

MINTY FENNEL

PASSIONATELY IMMUNE

PERKY PARSNIP

SIMPLY WHEATGRASS

VITAL MS SUPPORT

# Allergy Relief

MAKES ABOUT 16 OUNCES, 2 SERVINGS

▶ CALORIES: 72, FAT: 1 G, SUGAR: 14 G, PROTEIN: 2 G, CARBOHYDRATES: 22 G

*Allergies of all kinds can cause incredible discomfort, affecting the respiratory system, the sinuses, the skin, the eyes, and even the digestive system. Food can have a tremendous effect on the severity of allergies. One powerful allergy fighter is pineapple, which contains an enzyme that helps relieve sinus allergies in particular. Ginger is a great addition to this allergy-fighting juice because it is a natural antihistamine. Try this juice daily during allergy season.*

2 LEMONS
1 GREEN APPLE
1 LARGE ENGLISH CUCUMBER
½ CUP PARSLEY
ONE 1-INCH PIECE GINGER
TWO 1-INCH SLICES PINEAPPLE

Peel the lemons, leaving the pith, and cut them in half. Remove any seeds. Core the apple and cut it into chunks. Juice the lemons, apple, and cucumber. Push the parsley and ginger through the juicer with the pineapple. If your juicer instructions indicate that your machine cannot handle the skin and core, remove them from the pineapple before juicing. Stir to combine the juice before drinking.

**INGREDIENTS FOR RELIEVING ALLERGY SYMPTOMS:**

- Apple
- Asparagus
- Beet
- Blueberry
- Carrot
- Ginger
- Grape
- Green pepper
- Mango
- Onion
- Orange
- Raspberry
- Red pepper
- Strawberry
- Spinach
- Watercress

# Asparagus Arthritis Relief

MAKES ABOUT 24 OUNCES, 3 SERVINGS

▶ CALORIES: 60, FAT: 2 G, SUGAR: 8 G, PROTEIN: 2 G,
CARBOHYDRATES: 16 G

*Arthritis is characterized by pain, swelling, and inflammation in the joints. This juice should help soothe the suffering, because the ingredients target inflammation and pain. For example, the high amount of sulfur in asparagus can relieve joint swelling and pain. If you choose to use the olive oil in this juice, you will be benefiting from oleocanthal, which blocks the formation of inflammation-causing enzymes.*

1 APPLE
4 MEDIUM CARROTS
1 BROCCOLI STALK
4 LARGE CELERY STALKS
1 HANDFUL PARSLEY
5 ASPARAGUS SPEARS
1 TEASPOON EXTRA-VIRGIN OLIVE OIL (OPTIONAL)

Core and cut the apple into wedges. Cut the ends off the carrots. Juice the apple, broccoli, and carrots. Use the celery to push the parsley through the juicer. Juice the asparagus. Stir to blend the juices. Put 1 teaspoon olive oil (if using) in the bottom of a glass and pour the juice over. Stir to combine the juice and olive oil before drinking.

## INGREDIENTS FOR ARTHRITIS RELIEF:

- Apple
- Asparagus
- Avocado
- Bell pepper
- Broccoli
- Butternut squash
- Carrot

- Cherry
- Ginger
- Hot pepper
- Onion
- Parsley
- Passion fruit

# Breathe Easy

MAKES ABOUT 24 OUNCES, 3 SERVINGS

▶ CALORIES: 89, FAT: 0 G, SUGAR: 13 G, PROTEIN: 3 G, CARBOHYDRATES: 29 G

*Asthma is a chronic inflammatory disease. Asthma attacks can be dangerous; airways close off because they become inflamed, and the muscles that surround them tighten. This difficulty breathing can be improved with juices like Breathe Easy. The asthma-friendly food list is made up of fruits and vegetables that help lung function. This produce is rich in bioflavonoids like quercetin, found in apples, which can combat free radicals. Studies have shown that a healthy immune system is supported by selenium, beta-carotene, and vitamins A, C, and E, which are found in all the ingredients in this juice.*

2 GREEN APPLES
1 RED BELL PEPPER
1 SWEET POTATO
¼ LEMON
1 JICAMA
½ HEAD ENDIVE
1 CUP PARSLEY

Core the apples and cut them into quarters. Take the stem out of the bell pepper. Cut the sweet potato into wedges. Peel the lemon, leaving the pith, and cut it in half. Remove any visible seeds. Juice the apples, bell pepper, and jicama. Push the endive and parsley through the juicer with the sweet potato wedges. Juice the lemon. Stir to combine the juice before drinking.

## INGREDIENTS TO PREVENT OR RELIEVE ASTHMA:

- Apple
- Bell pepper
- Broccoli
- Carrot
- Endive
- Garlic
- Jicama
- Kiwi
- Lemon
- Lettuce
- Lime
- Orange
- Papaya
- Parsnip
- Pineapple
- Spinach
- Strawberry
- Sweet potato
- Tomato
- Watermelon
- Yellow onion

# Glowing Ginseng

MAKES ABOUT 16 OUNCES, 2 SERVINGS

▶ CALORIES: 70, FAT: 1 G, SUGAR: 12 G, PROTEIN: 3 G, CARBOHYDRATES: 20 G

*Chronic fatigue syndrome is a complicated illness that is characterized by many different symptoms, including fatigue, sore throat, impaired memory, muscle pain, joint pain, headaches, and insomnia. This glorious juice contains ingredients that can provide some relief. Ginseng can positively affect the immune system, which is often suppressed in this condition. Apricot and pumpkin are very high in beta-carotene, which fights the free radicals that cause inflammation and worsen chronic fatigue syndrome symptoms.*

1 CUP DICED PUMPKIN
1 RED BELL PEPPER
2 APRICOTS
½ LEMON
1 TEASPOON GINSENG POWDER

Remove the rind and seeds from the pumpkin and chop the flesh roughly. Remove the stem from the bell pepper. Pit the apricots. Peel the lemon, leaving the pith, and quarter it. Remove any seeds. Juice the pumpkin, bell pepper, apricots, and lemon. Stir the ginseng into the juice before drinking.

## INGREDIENTS TO FIGHT CHRONIC FATIGUE SYNDROME:

- Apricot
- Avocado
- Banana
- Beet
- Blueberry
- Broccoli
- Carrot
- Garlic
- Kale
- Kiwi
- Mango
- Orange
- Papaya
- Parsley
- Pumpkin
- Sweet potato
- Tomato

# Inflammation Buster

MAKES ABOUT 16 OUNCES, 2 SERVINGS

▶ CALORIES: 69, FAT: 0 G, SUGAR: 13 G, PROTEIN: 2 G, CARBOHYDRATES: 22 G

*We typically think of inflammation as a red area on the skin, perhaps around a bug bite or a wound that is not healing well. But inflammation is the body's system-wide response to anything it regards as damaging or irritating. It's a natural process when the body is trying to heal itself. But problems arise when the body turns on itself and inflammation becomes chronic. It can cause arthritis, asthma, allergies, heart disease, and even cancer. This pretty pink juice reduces inflammation, because the ingredients are high in antioxidants, carotenoids, and vitamins E and K.*

1 LEMON
1 ASIAN PEAR
1 BEET WITH GREENS
TWO ¾-INCH SLICES PINEAPPLE
ONE 1-INCH PIECE GINGER
PINCH OF GROUND NUTMEG
PINCH OF GROUND CINNAMON
PINCH OF GROUND CLOVES

Peel the lemon, leaving the pith, and quarter it. Remove any seeds. Cut the Asian pear into quarters. Juice the pear, beet, pineapple, lemon, and ginger. Stir the spices into the juice before drinking.

**INGREDIENTS TO REDUCE INFLAMMATION:**

- Apple
- Asparagus
- Avocado
- Bell pepper
- Blueberry
- Broccoli
- Carrot
- Cherry
- Garlic
- Ginger
- Hot pepper
- Kale
- Onion
- Parsley
- Spinach
- Strawberry

# Liquid Chlorophyll

MAKES ABOUT 20 OUNCES, 2 SERVINGS

▶ CALORIES: 95, FAT: 2 G, SUGAR: 15 G, PROTEIN: 5 G, CARBOHYDRATES: 45 G

*Cervical cancer is the second most common cancer in women, and like all other cancers, it can be affected by the food you eat and your lifestyle choices. Wheatgrass is a superfood that fights all types of cancer; its very high level of chlorophyll has been shown to reduce aflatoxins levels. Aflatoxins have been linked to the development of cervical cancer. Turmeric is a very good source of a phytochemical called curcumin that can protect the body from human papilloma virus, the most common cause of cervical cancer.*

1 GRANNY SMITH APPLE

1 SMALL HANDFUL WHEATGRASS

½ CUP ALFALFA SPROUTS

1 HANDFUL PARSLEY

5 LARGE CELERY STALKS

PINCH OF TURMERIC

Core and cut the apple into chunks. Chop the wheatgrass into 1-inch pieces. Juice the apple. Juice the wheatgrass, alfalfa sprouts, and parsley by pushing it through the juicer with the celery. Stir the turmeric into the juice before drinking.

**INGREDIENTS TO PREVENT CERVICAL CANCER:**

- Apple
- Blackberry
- Blueberry
- Broccoli
- Brussels sprout
- Cabbage
- Cauliflower
- Kale
- Kiwi
- Raspberry
- Strawberry
- Turmeric
- Wheatgrass

# Minty Fennel

MAKES ABOUT 24 OUNCES, 3 SERVINGS

▶ CALORIES: 82, FAT: 1 G, SUGAR: 5 G, PROTEIN: 4 G,
CARBOHYDRATES: 27 G

*Ulcerative colitis is an inflammatory disease of the digestive system, characterized by ulcers, abdominal pain, and chronic diarrhea. Diet can help control this condition. The ginger and fennel in this juice can reduce inflammation, which reduces the painful symptoms of this type of colitis.*

1 LEMON
1 FENNEL BULB WITH FRONDS
2 HANDFULS MINT
1 SMALL ENGLISH CUCUMBER
ONE ½-INCH PIECE GINGER

Peel the lemon, leaving the pith, and quarter it. Remove any seeds. Cut the fennel bulb into chunks and juice it. Juice the mint, using the cucumber to push the mint through the juicer. Juice the ginger and lemon. Stir to combine the juice before drinking.

# Perky Parsnip

MAKES ABOUT 24 OUNCES, 3 SERVINGS

▶ CALORIES: 80, FAT: 1 G, SUGAR: 8 G, PROTEIN: 3 G,
CARBOHYDRATES: 26 G

*Rheumatoid arthritis is an autoimmune disease that causes chronic inflammation in the joints, and sometimes in other areas of the body. It can flare up without warning and then subside. These flare-ups can be caused by diet, and this Perky Parsnip juice can help prevent them or minimize the severity. Fennel reduces inflammation system-wide and parsnip has been linked to pain relief.*

1 SMALL FENNEL BULB WITH FRONDS
1 LARGE PEAR
3 LARGE CELERY STALKS
1 HANDFUL PARSLEY
5 SPRIGS THYME
3 PARSNIPS

Cut the fennel bulb into chunks. Quarter the pear. Juice the fennel, celery, and pear. Push the parsley and thyme through the juicer with the parsnips. Stir to combine the juice before drinking.

**INGREDIENTS TO EASE AND PREVENT ULCERATIVE COLITIS:**

- Apple
- Blueberry
- Cucumber
- Fennel
- Garlic
- Ginger
- Grapefruit
- Honeydew
- Mango
- Mint
- Squash
- Zucchini

# Passionately Immune

▶ CALORIES: 92, FAT: 0 G, SUGAR: 6 G, PROTEIN: 2 G, CARBOHYDRATES: 28 G

*Inflammation is thought to be the cause of—or at least a contributor to—many chronic "lifestyle" diseases, including heart disease. Inflammation might be the missing piece to the puzzle of why some people have heart attacks and other people do not. Lifestyle factors such as exercise and diet play a huge role in the development of heart disease, but these factors also affect inflammation, so it is hard to separate them. This juice is a nice step forward to a healthier heart and less inflammation. Passion fruit is very rich in beta-carotene and B vitamins, which can lower cholesterol and blood pressure and improve blood circulation.*

1 GRANNY SMITH APPLE

1 SMALL ORANGE

1 SWEET POTATO

1 SMALL ENGLISH CUCUMBER

2 PASSION FRUITS

Core and chop the apple into chunks. Peel the orange, leaving the pith, and quarter it. Juice the sweet potato, cucumber, and apple. Cut the passion fruits in half, scoop the flesh into the juicer, and push it through with the orange. Stir to combine the juice before drinking.

## INGREDIENTS TO PREVENT AND EASE INFLAMMATIO

- Apple
- Asparagus
- Beet
- Bell pepper
- Broccoli
- Blueberry
- Carrot
- Celery
- Cranberry
- Garlic
- Grape
- Kale
- Onion
- Orange
- Passion fruit
- Raspberry
- Spinach
- Strawberry
- Sweet potato
- Tomato

## INGREDIENTS TO PREVENT AND EASE RHEUMATOID ARTHRITIS:

- Asparagus
- Avocado
- Beet
- Blueberry
- Broccoli
- Carrot
- Cranberry
- Cucumber
- Garlic
- Ginger
- Lemongrass
- Lettuce
- Peach
- Plum
- Pomegranate
- Red grape
- Spinach
- Strawberry
- Sweet potato
- Watercress

# Simply Wheatgrass

MAKES ABOUT 10 OUNCES, 1 SERVING

▶ CALORIES: 48, FAT: 0 G, SUGAR: 9 G, PROTEIN: 4 G,
CARBOHYDRATES: 18 G

*Fibromyalgia is a debilitating condition characterized by widespread pain in the muscles and bones combined with fatigue and memory problems. There is no cure for this condition, but the severity of the symptoms can be controlled with diet and juicing. Wheatgrass is a wonderful choice for fibromyalgia because it fights fatigue and is a nutritional powerhouse. The cabbage here is a nice base flavor, because it mellows out the intense taste of the wheatgrass.*

1 LEMON
½ HEAD WHITE CABBAGE
3½ OUNCES WHEATGRASS

Peel the lemon, leaving the pith, and quarter it. Remove any seeds. Chop the cabbage roughly. Chop the wheatgrass into 1-inch-long pieces. Juice the cabbage, wheatgrass, and lemon. Stir to combine the juice before drinking.

## INGREDIENTS TO EASE AND PREVENT ULCERATIVE COLITIS:

- Apple
- Blueberry
- Cucumber
- Fennel
- Garlic
- Ginger
- Grapefruit
- Honeydew
- Mango
- Mint
- Squash
- Zucchini

# Passionately Immune

▶ CALORIES: 92, FAT: 0 G, SUGAR: 6 G, PROTEIN: 2 G, CARBOHYDRATES: 28 G

*Inflammation is thought to be the cause of—or at least a contributor to—many chronic "lifestyle" diseases, including heart disease. Inflammation might be the missing piece to the puzzle of why some people have heart attacks and other people do not. Lifestyle factors such as exercise and diet play a huge role in the development of heart disease, but these factors also affect inflammation, so it is hard to separate them. This juice is a nice step forward to a healthier heart and less inflammation. Passion fruit is very rich in beta-carotene and B vitamins, which can lower cholesterol and blood pressure and improve blood circulation.*

1 GRANNY SMITH APPLE

1 SMALL ORANGE

1 SWEET POTATO

1 SMALL ENGLISH CUCUMBER

2 PASSION FRUITS

Core and chop the apple into chunks. Peel the orange, leaving the pith, and quarter it. Juice the sweet potato, cucumber, and apple. Cut the passion fruits in half, scoop the flesh into the juicer, and push it through with the orange. Stir to combine the juice before drinking.

**INGREDIENTS TO PREVENT AND EASE INFLAMMATION:**

- Apple
- Asparagus
- Beet
- Bell pepper
- Broccoli
- Blueberry
- Carrot
- Celery
- Cranberry
- Garlic
- Grape
- Kale
- Onion
- Orange
- Passion fruit
- Raspberry
- Spinach
- Strawberry
- Sweet potato
- Tomato

# Perky Parsnip

MAKES ABOUT 24 OUNCES, 3 SERVINGS

▶ CALORIES: 80, FAT: 1 G, SUGAR: 8 G, PROTEIN: 3 G,
CARBOHYDRATES: 26 G

*Rheumatoid arthritis is an autoimmune disease that causes chronic inflammation in the joints, and sometimes in other areas of the body. It can flare up without warning and then subside. These flare-ups can be caused by diet, and this Perky Parsnip juice can help prevent them or minimize the severity. Fennel reduces inflammation system-wide and parsnip has been linked to pain relief.*

1 SMALL FENNEL BULB WITH FRONDS
1 LARGE PEAR
3 LARGE CELERY STALKS
1 HANDFUL PARSLEY
5 SPRIGS THYME
3 PARSNIPS

Cut the fennel bulb into chunks. Quarter the pear. Juice the fennel, celery, and pear. Push the parsley and thyme through the juicer with the parsnips. Stir to combine the juice before drinking.

## INGREDIENTS TO PREVENT AND EASE RHEUMATOID ARTHRITIS:

- Asparagus
- Avocado
- Beet
- Blueberry
- Broccoli
- Carrot
- Cranberry
- Cucumber
- Garlic
- Ginger
- Lemongrass
- Lettuce
- Peach
- Plum
- Pomegranate
- Red grape
- Spinach
- Strawberry
- Sweet potato
- Watercress

# Simply Wheatgrass

MAKES ABOUT 10 OUNCES, 1 SERVING

▶ CALORIES: 48, FAT: 0 G, SUGAR: 9 G, PROTEIN: 4 G,
CARBOHYDRATES: 18 G

*Fibromyalgia is a debilitating condition characterized by widespread
pain in the muscles and bones combined with fatigue and memory
problems. There is no cure for this condition, but the severity of the
symptoms can be controlled with diet and juicing. Wheatgrass is a
wonderful choice for fibromyalgia because it fights fatigue and is a
nutritional powerhouse. The cabbage here is a nice base flavor, because
it mellows out the intense taste of the wheatgrass.*

1 LEMON
½ HEAD WHITE CABBAGE
3½ OUNCES WHEATGRASS

Peel the lemon, leaving the pith, and quarter it. Remove any seeds.
Chop the cabbage roughly. Chop the wheatgrass into 1-inch-long
pieces. Juice the cabbage, wheatgrass, and lemon. Stir to combine
the juice before drinking.

## INGREDIENTS TO EASE FIBROMYALGIA:

- Blueberry
- Broccoli
- Brussels sprout
- Cabbage
- Celery
- Cherry
- Garlic
- Ginger
- Grapefruit
- Green bell pepper
- Hot pepper
- Kale
- Kiwi
- Lemon
- Mango
- Orange
- Papaya
- Raspberry
- Red bell pepper
- Spinach
- Sweet potato
- Tomato

# Vital MS Support

▶ CALORIES: 82, FAT: 1 G, SUGAR: 10 G, PROTEIN: 4 G,
CARBOHYDRATES: 21 G

*Multiple sclerosis (MS) is an autoimmune disease, which means one's own immune system attacks itself—in this case, the central nervous system. MS is characterized by numbness, loss of balance, loss of muscle control, and vision problems. There is no cure for MS, but eating the right nutrients can make a difference in the progression and severity of the disease. Antioxidant-packed vegetables like beets, carrots, and kale can combat fatigue and reduce the risk of developing the painful bladder infections and constipation sometimes associated with MS.*

3 MEDIUM CARROTS

1 BEET WITH GREENS

1 GRANNY SMITH APPLE

2 LARGE CELERY STALKS

6 LARGE KALE LEAVES

4 STEMS CILANTRO

1 SMALL ENGLISH CUCUMBER

ONE 1-INCH PIECE GINGER

Cut the ends off the carrots. Core and cut the apple into wedges. Juice the beet, carrots, and celery. Juice the kale and cilantro by pushing it through with the cucumber. Juice the ginger and apple. Stir to combine the juice before drinking.

**INGREDIENTS TO COPE WITH MS:**

- Apple
- Beet
- Carrot
- Celery
- Cucumber
- Fennel

- Ginger
- Grape
- Kale
- Lemon
- Parsley
- Parsnip

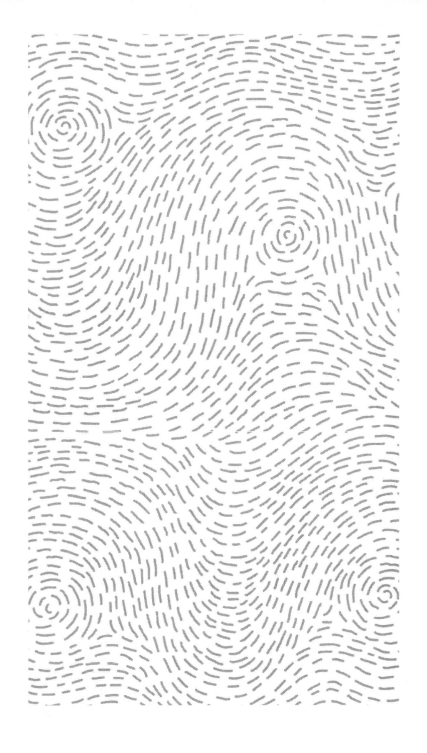

# CHAPTER ELEVEN

# Mind, Brain, and Mental Wellness

**APPLE ALZHEIMER'S PREVENTION**

**CLEARLY CABBAGE**

**FOCUS ON HYDRATION**

**HAPPY IN A GLASS**

**HEALTHFUL HEADACHE REMEDY**

**ROSY RELAXER**

**SWEET DREAMS**

# Apple Alzheimer's Prevention

MAKES ABOUT 32 OUNCES, 4 SERVINGS

▶ CALORIES: 56, FAT: 0 G, SUGAR: 12 G, PROTEIN: 1 G, CARBOHYDRATES: 18 G

*A great deal of research has been done in recent years, trying to pinpoint the exact causes of Alzheimer's disease. One thing that is apparent is that people with Alzheimer's have oxidative damage in the brain caused by free radicals. There are other factors for developing Alzheimer's, but juicing a variety of fruits and vegetables brimming with antioxidants can reduce cell damage from free radicals. Among all fruits and vegetables, apples contain the highest levels of an antioxidant called quercetin. This antioxidant protects the brain from cellular damage by free radicals, so a daily dose is a powerful preventive against Alzheimer's.*

1 LIME
3 MEDIUM APPLES
3 LARGE CELERY STALKS
1 SMALL ENGLISH CUCUMBER
ONE 1-INCH PIECE GINGER
4 SPRIGS THYME

Peel the lime, leaving the pith, and cut it into quarters. Remove any seeds. Core and cut the apples into quarters. Juice the apple and celery. Juice the cucumber, lime, ginger, and thyme. Stir to combine the juice before drinking.

## INGREDIENTS TO PREVENT ALZHEIMER'S DISEASE:

- Apple
- Avocado
- Beet
- Bell pepper
- Blackberry
- Blueberry
- Broccoli
- Brussels sprout
- Cabbage
- Cantaloupe
- Celery
- Garlic
- Grape
- Kale
- Mint
- Papaya
- Pear
- Plum
- Spinach
- Strawberry
- Sweet potato
- Watermelon

# Clearly Cabbage

MAKES ABOUT 28 OUNCES, 3 SERVINGS

▶ CALORIES: 66, FAT: 0 G, SUGAR: 12 G, PROTEIN: 2 G, CARBOHYDRATES: 21 G

*Being able to focus on a task that requires mental clarity can be difficult when you are tired, distracted, or your diet is less than optimal. This refreshing juice can help you concentrate and pay attention to the task at hand. The phytonutrients called anthocyanins in red cabbage have been linked to improved brain function. Make sure you get red cabbage for this juice, because the phytonutrients are in the substance that gives the cabbage its red color.*

2 MEDIUM GRANNY SMITH APPLES

3 LARGE CARROTS

1 LEMON

¼ HEAD RED CABBAGE

3 HANDFULS SPINACH

ONE 1-INCH PIECE GINGER

Core and cut the apples into chunks. Trim the ends off the carrots. Peel the lemon, leaving the pith, and cut it in half. Remove any seeds. Juice the apples and cabbage. Use the carrots to push the spinach through the juicer. Juice the ginger and lemon. Stir to combine the juice before drinking.

**INGREDIENTS FOR MENTAL CLARITY:**

- Apple
- Avocado
- Beet
- Blackberry
- Blueberry
- Broccoli
- Cabbage
- Cantaloupe
- Garlic
- Spinach
- Strawberry
- Sweet potato

# Focus on Hydration

MAKES ABOUT 16 OUNCES, 2 SERVINGS

▶ CALORIES: 122, FAT: 1 G, SUGAR: 27 G, PROTEIN: 2 G, CARBOHYDRATES: 34 G

*Sometimes the mental fog and confusion people suffer from is actually due to dehydration. The watermelon and cantaloupe in this refreshing juice is packed with water. The cantaloupe is doubly valuable for mental focus because its seeds contain a good amount of omega-3 fatty acids, which contribute to a healthy brain. Do not scoop out and discard the middle part of the melon that contains the seeds; simply juice it with the rest.*

TWO 1-INCH SLICES SEEDLESS WATERMELON

¼ CANTALOUPE

½ PAPAYA

½ CUP FRESH MINT LEAVES

1 TEASPOON CHLOROPHYLL

Cut the outer skin off the watermelon, leaving as much rind as possible. Cut the skin off the cantaloupe, leaving as much green as possible, and cut it into chunks, keeping the seeds. Peel and seed the papaya. Juice the watermelon and cantaloupe. Use the papaya to push the mint leaves through the juicer. Stir the chlorophyll into the juice before drinking.

**INGREDIENTS FOR HYDRATION AND BRAIN FOCUS:**

- Apple
- Avocado
- Beet
- Blackberry
- Blueberry
- Broccoli
- Cabbage
- Cantaloupe

- Cucumber
- Garlic
- Mint
- Papaya
- Spinach
- Strawberry
- Sweet potato
- Watermelon

# Happy in a Glass

▶ CALORIES: 43, FAT: 0 G, SUGAR: 3 G, PROTEIN: 2 G, CARBOHYDRATES: 14 G

*Most fresh juices are mood elevating because they are packed with nutrients that make the body happy. Studies have shown that deficiencies of vitamins $B_1$, $B_2$, $B_6$, $B_{12}$, C, and E can be linked to depression and anxiety, as can a lack of beta-carotene and magnesium. The combination of ingredients in this spicy juice addresses these deficiencies and boosts mood. Fennel is high in B vitamins, celery is a good source of magnesium, and carrot has beta-carotene.*

3 SMALL FENNEL BULBS WITH FRONDS
3 LARGE CARROTS
2 CELERY STALKS
½ ASIAN PEAR
ONE ½-INCH PIECE GINGER

Cut the fennel bulbs into chunks. Trim the ends off the carrots. Juice the fennel, carrots, celery, pear, and ginger. Stir to combine the juice before drinking.

## INGREDIENTS TO BOOST MOOD:

- Asparagus
- Bell pepper
- Broccoli
- Brussels sprout
- Cabbage
- Cantaloupe
- Carrot
- Cauliflower
- Celery
- Fennel
- Grapefruit

- Kale
- Mango
- Orange
- Papaya
- Peach
- Spinach
- Strawberry
- Tomato
- Watercress
- Watermelon

# Healthful Headache Remedy

MAKES ABOUT 24 OUNCES, 2 SERVINGS

▶  CALORIES: 49, FAT: 0 G, SUGAR: 9 G, PROTEIN: 1 G,
   CARBOHYDRATES: 16 G

*There are many things that can cause headaches, and hydration plays a role in relieving most of them. Fresh fruit and vegetable juices, as well as water, are wonderful ways of getting nutrients that combat headaches into your system quickly. Headaches, like many other health problems, can also be caused, in part, by toxins in the body. Often, when the body is detoxified, the pain will recede. Pears and carrots are very effective body cleansers.*

2 LARGE CARROTS
1 LARGE PEAR
3 LARGE CELERY STALKS
½ ENGLISH CUCUMBER
2 SPRIGS DILL

Trim the ends off the carrots. Quarter the pear. Juice the celery, carrots, pear, cucumber, and dill. Stir to combine the juice before drinking.

**INGREDIENTS TO PREVENT OR EASE HEADACHES:**

- Apple
- Avocado
- Beet
- Bell pepper
- Blackberry
- Blueberry
- Broccoli
- Brussels sprout
- Cabbage
- Cantaloupe
- Carrot
- Cauliflower
- Celery
- Cucumber
- Garlic
- Kale
- Mint
- Papaya
- Plum
- Spinach
- Strawberry
- Sweet potato
- Watercress
- Watermelon

# Rosy Relaxer

MAKES ABOUT 24 OUNCES, 3 SERVINGS

▶ CALORIES: 33, FAT: 1 G, SUGAR: 4 G, PROTEIN: 2 G, CARBOHYDRATES: 10 G

*Anxiety creates a sense of fear, worry, and dread. Although there is a psychological element, there can also be a nutritional component, as well. Juicing can provide food therapy for anxiety by combining ingredients that promote calm. Anxiety can be caused or worsened by a folic acid deficiency, and asparagus is a fabulous source of this nutrient. Other B vitamins can eliminate or lessen the impact of anxiety, and can be found in the lemon and parsley in this juice.*

1 LARGE LEMON
3 PLUM TOMATOES
1 SMALL RED BELL PEPPER
1 LARGE ENGLISH CUCUMBER
1 HANDFUL PARSLEY
6 ASPARAGUS STALKS
½ GARLIC CLOVE

Peel the lemon, leaving the pith, and quarter it. Remove any seeds. Juice the tomatoes and bell pepper. Use the cucumber to push the parsley through the juicer. Add the lemon, asparagus, and garlic to the juicer. Stir to combine the juice before drinking.

## INGREDIENTS TO CALM ANXIETY:

- Apple
- Apricot
- Asparagus
- Avocado
- Blackberry
- Blueberry
- Cantaloupe
- Cauliflower
- Fennel
- Grapes
- Limes
- Orange
- Parsnip
- Peach
- Pear
- Pineapple
- Spinach
- Strawberry
- Tomato

# Sweet Dreams

MAKES ABOUT 16 OUNCES, 2 SERVINGS

▶ CALORIES: 71, FAT: 1 G, SUGAR: 15 G, PROTEIN: 2 G,
CARBOHYDRATES: 23 G

*Everyone occasionally has a restless night. But when this problem becomes chronic, it takes a serious toll on the body. The complex carbohydrates in carrots and celery stimulate serotonin production and promote sleep. Watercress is also a wonderful choice for preventing insomnia because it contains an amino acid that boosts the production of hormones that are low in people suffering from insomnia.*

1 GRANNY SMITH APPLE

1 LARGE CARROT

¼ LEMON

4 LARGE CELERY STALKS

1 CUP WATERCRESS

1 CUP PARSLEY

¼ TEASPOON GROUND NUTMEG

Core and cut the apple into chunks. Cut the end off the carrot. Peel the lemon, leaving the pith, and cut it in half. Remove any visible seeds. Put the apple through the juicer with the carrot. Use the celery to push the watercress and parsley through the juicer. Juice the lemon. Stir the nutmeg into the juice before drinking.

## INGREDIENTS TO PREVENT INSOMNIA:

- Alfalfa sprouts
- Avocado
- Banana
- Bean sprouts
- Beet
- Carrot
- Celery
- Green apple
- Lettuce
- Pineapple
- Plum
- Tomato
- Watercress

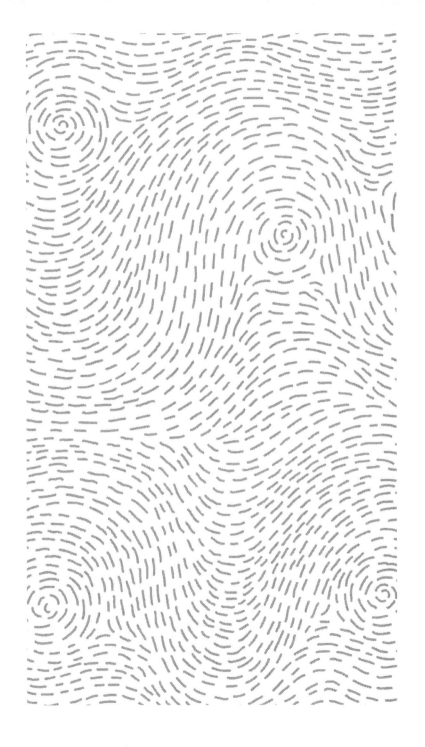

# CHAPTER TWELVE

# Beauty and Skin Enhancers

BEETING ECZEMA

CARROT CLEAR-UP

CIRCLE BANISHER

CITRUS CELLULITE
BE GONE

LOTS OF LOCKS

SHINY TRESSES

VANISHING VEINS

# Beeting Eczema

▶ CALORIES: 76, FAT: 1 G, SUGAR: 12 G, PROTEIN: 3 G, CARBOHYDRATES: 23 G

*Eczema is a painful skin condition characterized by blistered, flaking, itchy skin. Luckily, symptoms can be lessened and even prevented with proper nutrition. The carrots and ginger in this recipe can combat chronic inflammation, which is linked to eczema flare-ups. The beets are very rich in nutrients that can help protect the skin.*

6 MEDIUM CARROTS

2 LEMONS

4 LARGE BEETS WITH GREENS

6 CELERY STALKS

1 HANDFUL PARSLEY

ONE 2-INCH PIECE GINGER

Cut the ends off the carrots. Peel the lemons, leaving the pith, and quarter them. Remove any seeds. Juice the beets and carrots. Use the celery to push the parsley through the juicer. Juice the ginger and lemons. Stir to combine the juice before drinking.

## INGREDIENTS TO PREVENT AND EASE ECZEMA:

- Apple
- Asparagus
- Avocado
- Blueberry
- Carrot
- Celery
- Cranberry
- Cucumber
- Lime
- Parsley
- Spinach
- Tomato
- Watercress
- Watermelon

# Carrot Clear-Up

MAKES ABOUT 24 OUNCES, 3 SERVINGS

▶ CALORIES: 82, FAT: 1 G, SUGAR: 7 G, PROTEIN: 4 G, CARBOHYDRATES: 20 G

*People used to think oily food and chocolate caused acne, but we now know that these foods don't cause breakouts. However, eating a healthier diet can clear up your skin. Carrot Clear-Up juice is a wonderful blend of skin-clearing nutrients. Carrots are high in beta-carotene, vitamin A, and antioxidants that prevent skin damage and maintain the skin's suppleness. Kale is also high in beta-carotene, which protects against free radicals. Apples and celery are packed with magnesium, vitamins C and E, and B vitamins, which all support clear, lovely skin.*

1 GRANNY SMITH APPLE

3 MEDIUM CARROTS

1 CUP CHOPPED KALE

1 CELERY STALK

1 CUP BROCCOLI FLORETS

2 SPRIGS CILANTRO

Core and cut the apple into chunks. Cut the ends off the carrots. Juice the apple and use 1 carrot to push the kale through the juicer. Juice the remaining 2 carrots, celery, broccoli, and cilantro. Stir to combine the juice before drinking.

**INGREDIENTS TO PREVENT AND HEAL ACNE:**

- Apple
- Beet
- Cantaloupe
- Carrot
- Cilantro
- Cucumber
- Endive
- Green apple
- Kale
- Kiwi
- Lettuce
- Spinach
- Tomato
- Watercress
- Watermelon

# Circle Banisher

▶ CALORIES: 38, FAT: 0 G, SUGAR: 10 G, PROTEIN: 2 G,
CARBOHYDRATES: 16 G

*Black circles under the eyes may be the result of aging or genetics, but sometimes seasonal allergies, vitamin deficiency, or inflammation play a part. These circles can be improved by diet. Apples are packed with antioxidants that can help flush toxins from the body, improving the look under the eyes. Fennel is a diuretic, so it can decrease the puffiness under the eyes, minimizing the look of dark circles. Beets are very high in iron, which reduces the severity of the dark circles.*

¼ LEMON
2 GRANNY SMITH APPLES
6 OR 7 SPINACH LEAVES
1 SMALL ENGLISH CUCUMBER
2 BEETS WITH GREENS
¼ BULB FENNEL WITH FRONDS
1 CUP PARSLEY
5 SPRIGS THYME

Peel the lemon, leaving the pith, and cut it in half. Remove any visible seeds. Core and cut the apples into chunks. Juice the apple. Add the spinach leaves and use the cucumber to push them through the juicer. Juice the beets, fennel, parsley, thyme, and lemon. Stir to combine the juice before drinking.

**INGREDIENTS TO CLEAR UP DARK CIRCLES:**

- Avocado
- Beet
- Blueberry
- Collard greens
- Fennel
- Kiwi
- Orange
- Pear
- Spinach
- Strawberry

# Citrus Cellulite Be Gone

MAKES ABOUT 16 OUNCES, 2 SERVINGS

▶ CALORIES: 88, FAT: 0 G, SUGAR: 20 G, PROTEIN: 2 G,
CARBOHYDRATES: 27 G

*Cellulite is unsightly dimpling under the skin. It is most common in areas where people tend to have fat deposits, such as the thighs, and is the result of this fatty tissue getting caught in the fibrous cords that connect the skin to the underlying muscle. Flushing the toxins from your body can help smooth your skin, and juicing can be part of the answer. Drinking a lot of water, along with fresh fruit juices, may help get rid of or reduce cellulite. Citrus fruits, such as grapefruit, oranges, and limes, are packed with bioflavonoids. These nutrients can prevent the characteristic orange peel effect of cellulite by strengthening the capillaries.*

1 LARGE RUBY-RED GRAPEFRUIT
2 LARGE ORANGES
½ LIME
ONE 1-INCH PIECE GINGER ROOT

Peel the grapefruit, oranges, and lime, leaving the pith. Remove the seeds from the lime, because they will make the juice bitter. Cut the grapefruit and oranges into quarters. Juice the grapefruit, oranges, lime, and ginger. Stir to combine the juice before serving.

## INGREDIENTS FOR REDUCING CELLULITE:

- Apple
- Cabbage
- Carrot
- Celery
- Cucumber
- Endive
- Fennel

- Grapefruit
- Lemon
- Lime
- Orange
- Parsley
- Tomato
- Watercress

# Lots of Locks

▶ CALORIES: 49, FAT: 1 G, SUGAR: 7 G, PROTEIN: 4 G, CARBOHYDRATES: 13 G

*If you are not exercising, eating a balanced diet rich in nutrients, and getting enough sleep, your crowning glory will reflect those deficiencies by being thin and dull. Spinach is full of omega-3 fatty acids and vitamin A, both of which help hair grow stronger and prevent hair loss. The broccoli in this juice is a great source of vitamin C, which can prevent breakage, and the carrot helps purge toxins from the body, which can slow hair growth. This juice will make your hair glorious from the inside out.*

1 LARGE CARROT
1 CUP CHOPPED SPINACH
1 CUP BROCCOLI FLORETS
2 BRUSSELS SPROUTS
¼ SMALL RED ONION
1 BEET WITH GREENS

Cut the end off the carrot. Juice the spinach, broccoli, Brussels sprouts, carrot, onion, and beet. Stir to combine the juice before drinking.

## INGREDIENTS FOR THICK, HEALTHY HAIR:

- Asparagus
- Avocado
- Banana
- Beet
- Blueberry
- Broccoli
- Brussels sprout
- Carrot
- Cilantro
- Collard greens
- Green bean
- Kale
- Onion
- Spinach
- Sweet potato
- Tomato
- Watermelon

# Shiny Tresses

MAKES ABOUT 28 OUNCES, 3 SERVINGS

▶ CALORIES: 64, FAT: 0 G, SUGAR: 9 G, PROTEIN: 2 G, CARBOHYDRATES: 19 G

*Beautiful, healthy hair is a direct reflection of a healthy, nourished body. Beta-carotene can prevent dull hair and dandruff, and it is found in sweet potatoes. Swiss chard is packed with vitamins A and C, which increase sebum, hair's natural conditioner.*

1 LEMON
1 LARGE ORANGE
4 SMALL CARROTS
10 LARGE RIPE STRAWBERRIES
1 LARGE SWEET POTATO
6 LARGE SWISS CHARD LEAVES

Peel the lemon and orange, leaving the pith. Remove the seeds from the lemon. Cut the ends off the carrots. Hull the strawberries. Cut the lemon, orange, and sweet potato into quarters. Juice the Swiss chard, pushing it through the juicer with the lemon and orange wedges. Juice the sweet potato, carrots, and strawberries. Stir to combine the juice before drinking.

**INGREDIENTS FOR SHINY HAIR:**

- Asparagus
- Avocado
- Banana
- Blueberry
- Broccoli
- Carrot
- Cilantro
- Collard greens
- Green bean
- Kale
- Spinach
- Sweet potato
- Tomato
- Watermelon

# Vanishing Veins

MAKES ABOUT 16 OUNCES, 2 SERVINGS

▶ CALORIES: 94, FAT: 0 G, SUGAR: 9 G, PROTEIN: 2 G,
CARBOHYDRATES: 26 G

*Varicose veins are unattractive and in some cases uncomfortable. They appear when the valves in the veins that move the blood through the legs are weakened, causing pooling. There are many causes of varicose veins, from obesity to sitting for long periods of time. The best way to prevent varicose veins is to drink lots of water, keep moving, and include fruits and vegetables as part of your diet, either whole or in refreshing juices. Vegetables like beets can keep the veins and arteries elastic, which helps prevent varicose veins. Pineapple is also effective for preventing this problem, as it tends to dissolve fibrin, a protein that can disrupt the flow of blood.*

¼ LEMON

½ SMALL PINEAPPLE

½ YELLOW BELL PEPPER

1 MEDIUM BEET WITH GREENS

3 CELERY STALKS

ONE ½-INCH PIECE GINGER

Peel the lemon, leaving the pith, and cut it in half. Remove any visible seeds. Cut the pineapple into chunks, leaving the skin and the core. Check your juicer instructions to see if it can handle this part of the pineapple, and if not, peel and core the fruit. Take the stem out of the bell pepper. Juice the beet, pineapple, celery, bell pepper, lemon, and ginger. Stir to combine the juice before drinking.

**INGREDIENTS TO PREVENT VARICOSE VEINS:**

- Beet
- Bell pepper
- Blackberry
- Black currant
- Blueberry
- Celery
- Cherry
- Cranberry
- Garlic
- Grape
- Grapefruit
- Kale
- Kiwi
- Lemon
- Orange
- Pineapple
- Spinach

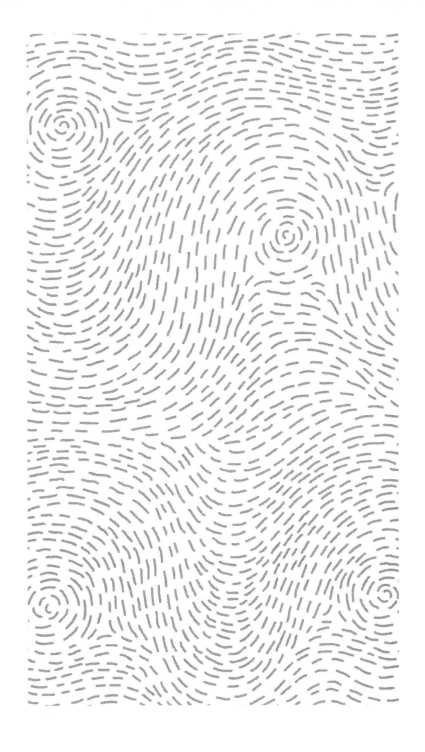

# References

Balch, Phyllis A. *Prescription for Dietary Wellness: Using Foods to Heal.* 2nd ed. New York: Avery, 2003.

Balch, Phyllis A. *Prescription for Nutritional Healing: A Practical A-to-Z Reference to Drug-Free Remedies Using Vitamins, Minerals, Herbs, and Food Supplements.* 5th ed. New York: Avery, 2010.

Colbin, Annemarie. *Food and Healing.* New York: Ballantine Books, 1986.

Collier Cool, Lisa. "Inflammation: The Root Cause of All Disease?" Yahoo Health. January 16, 2013. http://health.yahoo.net/experts/dayinhealth/inflammation-root-cause-all-disease.

Ehrlich, Steven D. "Chronic Fatigue Syndrome." University of Maryland Medical Center. Last modified May 31, 2013. http://umm.edu/health/medical/altmed/condition/chronic-fatigue-syndrome.

Environmental Working Group. "All 48 Fruits and Vegetables with Pesticide Residue Data." Accessed December 10, 2013. http://www.ewg.org/foodnews/list.php.

Haas, Elson M., and Buck Levin. *Staying Healthy with Nutrition: The Complete Guide to Diet and Nutritional Medicine.* rev. ed. Berkeley, CA: Celestial Arts, 2006.

Haas, Elson M., and Daniella Chace. *The Detox Diet: The Definitive Guide for Lifelong Vitality with Recipes, Menus, and Detox Plans.* 3rd ed. New York: Ten Speed Press, 2012.

Hendrick, Bill. "Beet Juice Good for Brain." WebMD. November 3, 2010. http://www.webmd.com/brain/news/20101103/beet-juice-good-for-brain.

Holford, Patrick. *The New Optimum Nutrition Bible.* rev. ed. New York: Crossing Press, 2004.

Howell, Edward. *Enzyme Nutrition.* New York: Avery Publishing, 1985.

Kendall-Reed, Penny, and Stephen Reed. *Healing Arthritis: Complementary Naturopathic, Orthopedic, and Drug Treatments.* Toronto: CCNM Press, 2004.

Murray, Michael T. *Diabetes and Hypoglycemia: Your Natural Guide to Healing with Diet, Vitamins, Minerals, Herbs, Exercise, and Other Natural Methods.* New York: Three Rivers Press, 1994.

Murray, Michael T., and Joseph Pizzorno. *The Encyclopedia of Natural Medicine.* 3rd ed. New York: Atria Paperback, 2012.

Nelson, Jennifer K. "Is Juicing Healthier Than Eating Whole Fruits or Vegetables?" Mayo Clinic. Accessed November 28, 2013. http://www.mayoclinic.com/health/juicing/AN02107.

Nestle, Marion. *What to Eat.* New York: North Point Press, 2006.

Nguyen, Anna. "Juicing: How Healthy Is It?" WebMD. Last modified January 11, 2012. http://www.webmd.com/diet/features/juicing-health-risks-and-benefits.

Nutrition Source. "Vegetables and Fruits." Harvard School of Public Health. Accessed December 3, 2013. http://www.hsph.harvard.edu/nutritionsource/what-should-you-eat/vegetables-and-fruits.

Nutrition Source. "Vegetables and Fruits: Get Plenty Every Day." Harvard School of Public Health. Accessed December 3, 2013. http://www.hsph.harvard.edu/nutritionsource/vegetables-full-story.

Rowland, David W. *The Nutritional Bypass: Reverse Atherosclerosis Without Surgery.* Parry Sound, ON: Rowland Publications, 1995.

Subramanian, Sushma. "Fact or Fiction: Raw Veggies Are Healthier Than Cooked Ones." *Scientific American.* March 31, 2009. http://www.scientificamerican.com/article.cfm?id=raw-veggies-are-healthier.

University of Michigan Health System. "Healing Foods Pyramid." Accessed December 6, 2013. http://www.med.umich.edu/umim/food-pyramid/fruits_and_vegetables.htm.

Walters, Sheryl. "Chlorophyll in Wheatgrass Proven to Fight Cancer." NaturalNews.com. June 10, 2009. http://www.naturalnews.com/026418_chlorophyll_wheatgrass_skin.html.

Walters, Sheryl. "Raw Food Diet Offers Considerable Benefits." NaturalNews.com. May 10, 2009. http://www.naturalnews.com/026238_food_diet_raw.html.

Wood, Rebecca. *The New Whole Foods Encyclopedia: A Comprehensive Resource for Healthy Eating.* rev. ed. New York: Penguin Books, 2010.

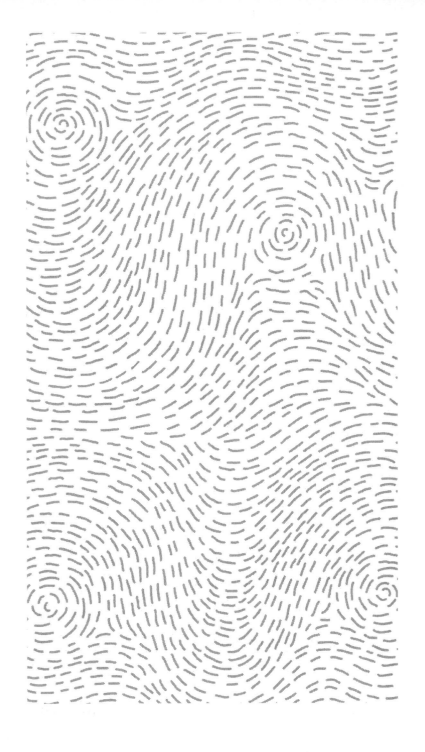

# Index

## A

Achy Breaky Muscles,
78–79
Acid Away, 136–137
Acne, 54, 242
ingredients to prevent
and heal, 243
Aftermath Recovery,
182–183
Alfalfa sprouts
Liquid Chlorophyll,
210
Allergies, 200, 208
ingredients for
relieving symptoms,
201
sinus, 200
Allergy Relief, 200–201
Allspice, 48
Alzheimer's disease,
54, 224
ingredients to
prevent, 225
Androsterone, 106
Anemia, 54, 94
ingredients for
preventing, 95
Anthocyanins, 226
Anti-aging, 54
Antioxidants, 7, 8
Anxiety, 234
ingredients to calm,
235
Apple Alzheimer's
Prevention, 224–225
Apples, 21, 47, 120

Achy Breaky
Muscles, 78
Acid Away, 136
Allergy Relief, 200
Apple Alzheimer's
Prevention, 224
Asparagus Arthritis
Relief, 202
Beet Cramps, 82
Beet the Heat, 84
Breathe Easy, 204
Bye-Bye Nausea, 138
Carrot Clear-Up, 242
Carrot Colon
Cleanse, 88
Circle Banisher, 244
Clean Artery
Sweep, 92
Clearly Cabbage, 226
Cutting Cancer, 166
Does a Body
Good, 140
Easy Digestion, 142
Flu Fighter, 122
Full System Boost, 124
Get Things
Moving, 144
Good Morning, 146
Gout Be Gone, 168
Gut Flora Builder, 150
Before Gym Blitz, 184
Healthful Heart
Ginger, 172
Healthy Heart
Summer Salad, 112
Healthy Prostate
Blend, 104–105

IBS Support, 152
LDL Reducer, 102
Liquid Chlorophyll,
210
Meal in a Glass, 154
Metabolism Mover,
156
Passionately
Immune, 214
Pick Me Up, 192
Ready to Recover, 194
Slow Energy, 196
Spinach Sugar
Stabilizer, 108
Splendid Sinuses, 132
Superfood Detox, 120
Sweet Dreams, 236
Thyroid Buddy, 178
Vital MS Support, 220
Apple seeds, 14
Apricots, 22
Glowing Ginseng, 206
Arteriosclerosis, 92
ingredients to
prevent, 93
Arthritis, 54, 202, 208
ingredients for relief
of, 203
Asparagus, 33
Asparagus Arthritis
Relief, 202
Rosy Relaxer, 234
Asparagus Arthritis Relief,
202–203
Asthma, 54, 204, 208
ingredients to prevent
or relieve, 205

Avocado, 22
    Ready to Recover, 194
Ayurveda, 5

# B

Balancing Act, 80–81
Bananas, 23
    Ready to Recover, 194
Basil, 48
    Garden Fresh Blast, 94
    Promote Prostate
        Health, 174
Beat Breast Cancer,
    176–177
Beauty and skin
    enhancers, 240–253
    Beeting Eczema,
        240–241
    Carrot Clear-Up,
        242–243
    Circle Banisher,
        244–245
    Citrus Cellulite Be
        Gone, 246–247
    Lots of Locks,
        248–249
    Shiny Tresses,
        250–251
    Vanishing Veins,
        252–253
Beet Cramps, 82–83
Beeting Eczema, 240–241
Beets, 34, 120
    Balancing Act, 80
    Beet Cramps, 82
    Beeting Eczema, 240
    Beet the Heat, 84
    Better Body, 162
    Carrot Colon
        Cleanse, 88
    Circle Banisher, 244
    Get Things
        Moving, 144
    Healthy Heart
        Summer Salad, 112

Heart Beet, 100
Inflammation
    Buster, 208
    Kick the Cold, 128
    Lots of Locks, 248
    Meal in a Glass, 154
    Metabolism Mover,
        156
    Superfood Detox, 120
    Vanishing Veins, 252
    Vital MS Support, 220
Beet the Heat, 84–85
Beet with greens, 10
Before Gym Blitz, 184–185
Bell peppers, 34. See also
    Green bell peppers;
    Orange bell peppers;
    Red bell peppers
Berries. See Blackberries;
    Blueberries;
    Cranberries;
    Raspberries;
    Strawberries
Beta-carotene, 126, 166,
    188, 204, 206, 214, 230,
    242, 250
Betacyanins, 162
Better Body, 162–163
Bioflavonoids,, 204
Blackberries, 23
    Aftermath Recovery,
        182
    Bonny Bone Fruit
        Surprise, 164
Bladder Infection Be
    Gone, 86–87
Bloating, ingredients to
    soothe, 159
Blood sugar, ingredients
    to stabilize, 109
Blueberries, 23, 47
    Bladder Infection Be
        Gone, 86
    Carrot Colon
        Cleanse, 88

Clean as a Whistle
    Kidney Cleanse, 90
    Does a Body Good, 140
    Promote Prostate
        Health, 174
Bok choy, 34–35
Bone health, 54
Bonny Bone Fruit
    Surprise, 164–165
Brain focus, ingredients
    for, 229
Breast cancer, 176
    ingredients to
        fight, 177
Breathe Easy, 204–205
Broccoli, 35
    Aftermath Recovery,
        182
    Asparagus Arthritis
        Relief, 202
    Carrot Clear-Up, 242
    Carrot Colon
        Cleanse, 88
    Clean Artery Sweep, 92
    Green Heartburn
        Relief, 148
    Green Joint Relief, 98
    Healthy Prostate
        Blend, 104–105
    Lots of Locks, 248
    Meal in a Glass, 154
    Ready to Recover, 194
    Spinach Sugar
        Stabilizer, 108
Bromelain, 130
Brussels Sprouts, 35–36
    Getting a Boost, 126
    Healthy Prostate
        Blend, 104–105
    Lots of Locks, 248
    Meal in a Glass, 154
Burn, Baby, Burn, 186–187
Butternut squash, 36
Butylphthalide, 102
Bye-Bye Nausea, 138–139

# C

Cabbage, 36
    Acid Away, 136
    Clearly Cabbage, 226
    Does a Body Good, 140
    Papaya Gut
        Reprieve, 158
    Simply Wheatgrass,
        218
Caffeine, 16
Calcium, 164
Cancer, 54, 208
    breast, 176–177
    colon, 88, 170–171
    ingredients to help
        prevent, 167
    prostate, 104, 174–175
Cancer and disease
    prevention, 162–179
    Beat Breast Cancer,
        176–177
    Better Body, 162–163
    Bonny Bone Fruit
        Surprise, 164–165
    Cutting Cancer,
        166–167
    Gout Be Gone, 168–169
    Happy Colon, 170–171
    Healthful Heart
        Ginger, 172–173
    Promote Prostate
        Health, 174–175
    Thyroid Buddy,
        178–179
Cantaloupe, 24
    Focus on
        Hydration, 228
Carotenoids, 166
Carrot Clear-Up, 242–243
Carrot Colon Cleanse,
    88–89
Carrots, 10, 37, 120
    Asparagus Arthritis
        Relief, 202

Balancing Act, 80
Beet Cramps, 82
Beeting Eczema, 240
Beet the Heat, 84
Better Body, 162
Bye-Bye Nausea, 138
Carrot Clear-Up, 242
Carrot Colon
    Cleanse, 88
Clean Artery
    Sweep, 92
Clearly Cabbage, 226
Cutting Cancer, 166
Easy Digestion, 142
Fat Furnace, 188
Flu Fighter, 122
Full System
    Boost, 124
Garden Fresh
    Blast, 94
Get Things
    Moving, 144
Getting a Boost, 126
Good Morning, 146
Gout Be Gone, 168
Green Heartburn
    Relief, 148
Gut Flora
    Builder, 150
Happy in a Glass, 230
Healthful Headache
    Remedy, 232
Healthy Heart
    Summer Salad, 112
Heart Beet, 100
Lots of Locks, 248
Love Boost, 106
Meal in a Glass, 154
Pick Me Up, 192
Under Pressure, 114
Shiny Tresses, 250
Spinach Sugar
    Stabilizer, 108
Superfood Detox, 120
Sweet Dreams, 236

Vital MS Support, 220
Cauliflower, 37
    Does a Body Good, 140
    Meal in a Glass, 154
Cayenne pepper, 49
    Citrus Cough
        Buster, 118
    Clean as a Whistle
        Kidney Cleanse, 90
Celery, 10, 37–38, 47
    Achy Breaky
        Muscles, 78
    Acid Away, 136
    Apple Alzheimer's
        Prevention, 224
    Asparagus Arthritis
        Relief, 202
    Beeting Eczema, 240
    Beet the Heat, 84
    Better Body, 162
    Bladder Infection Be
        Gone, 86
    Carrot Clear-Up, 242
    Clean Artery
        Sweep, 92
    Easy Digestion, 142
    Fat Furnace, 188
    Flu Fighter, 122
    Garden Fresh
        Blast, 94
    Getting a Boost, 126
    Gout Be Gone, 168
    Green Go-Go, 190
    Green Heartburn
        Relief, 148
    Gut Flora
        Builder, 150
    Happy in a Glass, 230
    Healthful Headache
        Remedy, 232
    Healthful Heart
        Ginger, 172
    Heart Beet, 100
    IBS Support, 152
    LDL Reducer, 102

Liquid Chlorophyll, 210
Love Boost, 106
Perky Parsnip, 216
Pick Me Up, 192
Under Pressure, 114
Slow Energy, 196
Stimulating Sunshine, 110
Sweet Dreams, 236
Vanishing Veins, 252
Vital MS Support, 220
Cellulite, 246
ingredients for reducing, 247
Centrifugal juicers, 9–10
Cervical cancer, 210
ingredients to prevent, 211
Cherries, 24, 47
Gout Be Gone, 168
Ready to Recover, 194
Cherry tomatoes, 47
Chlorophyll, 210
Focus on Hydration, 228
Cholesterol, ingredients to lower, 103, 113
Chromium, 194
Chronic fatigue syndrome, 206
Cilantro, 49
Carrot Clear-Up, 242
Cutting Cancer, 166
Before Gym Blitz, 184
IBS Support, 152
Vital MS Support, 220
Cinnamon, 50
Inflammation Buster, 208
Ready to Recover, 194
Spinach Sugar Stabilizer, 108
Circle Banisher, 244–245

Citrus Cellulite Be Gone, 246–247
Citrus Cough Buster, 118–119
Clean Artery Sweep, 92–93
Clean as a Whistle Kidney Cleanse, 90–91
Clearly Cabbage, 226–227
Cloves, 50
Inflammation Buster, 208
Cognitive function, 8
Colds, 128
ingredients for fighting the common, 129
Collard greens, 38, 47
Cutting Cancer, 166
Green Heartburn Relief, 148
Colon
ingredients for cleansing, 89
mucus in, 88
Colon cancer, 88, 170
ingredients to prevent, 171
Confusion, 228
Constipation, 54, 144
ingredients to ease, 145
Corn
Burn, Baby, Burn, 186
Coughs, ingredients for combating, 119
Cranberries, 25, 86
Bladder Infection Be Gone, 86
Citrus Cough Buster, 118
Happy Colon, 170
Thyroid Buddy, 178
Cucumbers, 10, 38–39, 47. See also English cucumber

Aftermath Recovery, 182
Green Heartburn Relief, 148
Spinach Sugar Stabilizer, 108
Cumin, 50
Curcumin, 210
Cutting Cancer, 166–167

D
Dark circles, 244
ingredients to clear up, 245
Detoxing, 59
avoiding caffeine in, 16
Diabetes, 108
juicing and, 16
Digestion, 7
ingredients to aid, 143
problems with, 54
Digestion Enhancers. See Weight loss and digestion enhancers
Dill
Healthful Headache Remedy, 232
D-mannose, 86
Doctor, consulting your, 62
Does a Body Good, 140–141

E
Easy Digestion, 142–143
Eczema, 240
ingredients to prevent and ease, 241
Endive, 39
Breathe Easy, 204
Energy and vitality boost, 182–197
Aftermath Recovery, 182–183

Burn, Baby, Burn,
    186–187
Fat Furnace, 188–189
Green Go-Go,
    190–191
Before Gym Blitz,
    184–185
Pick Me Up, 192–193
Ready to Recover,
    194–195
Slow Energy, 196–197
English cucumber
Achy Breaky
    Muscles, 78
Acid Away, 136
Allergy Relief, 200
Apple Alzheimer's
    Prevention, 224
Beet Cramps, 82
Burn, Baby, Burn, 186
Bye-Bye Nausea, 138
Circle Banisher, 244
Clean Artery
    Sweep, 92
Does a Body Good, 140
Flu Fighter, 122
Garden Fresh Blast, 94
Gout Be Gone, 168
Green Go-Go, 190
Healthful Headache
    Remedy, 232
Healthful Heart
    Ginger, 172
Healthy Prostate
    Blend, 104–105
Heart Beet, 100
Kick the Cold, 128
LDL Reducer, 102
Love Boost, 106
Metabolism Mover,
    156
Minty Fennel, 212
Passionately
    Immune, 214
Pick Me Up, 192

Under Pressure, 114
Rosy Relaxer, 234
Stimulating
    Sunshine, 110
Superfood Detox, 120
Vital MS Support, 220
Estrogen, 80
Exercise, juice cleanse
    and, 17, 64

F

Fasting, 15, 59
Fat, ingredients to
    burn, 189
Fat Furnace, 188–189
Fatigue, 54
    ingredients to
        combat, 193
Fennel, 39, 142
    Circle Banisher, 244
    Easy Digestion, 142
    Gut Flora Builder, 150
    Happy in a Glass, 230
    Minty Fennel, 212
    Perky Parsnip, 216
    Thyroid Buddy, 178
Fiber, 6, 7
Fibromyalgia, 218
    ingredients to
        ease, 219
Figs, 25
Flavonoids, 166
Flaxseed oil
    Great Grapefruit
        Cleanse, 96
Flu, 122
    ingredients for
        fighting, 123
Flu Fighter, 122–123
Focus on Hydration,
    228–229
Folic acid deficiency, 234
Free radicals, 8, 224, 242
Fruit juice, versus
    vegetable juice, 20–21

Fruits, 21–33. *See
    also specific*
    eating, 13
Full System Boost,
    124–125

G

Garden Fresh Blast, 94–95
Garlic, 39–40
    Full System Boost, 124
    Great Grapefruit
        Cleanse, 96
    Gut Flora Builder, 150
    Healthy Heart
        Summer Salad, 112
    Kick the Cold, 128
    Rosy Relaxer, 234
Gas, ingredients to
    soothe, 159
Gastroesophageal reflux
    disease (GERD), 136
    ingredients for
        preventing, 137
General health and well-
    being, 78–115
    Achy Breaky Muscles,
        78–79
    Balancing Act, 80–81
    Beet Cramps, 82–83
    Beet the Heat, 84–85
    Bladder Infection Be
        Gone, 86–87
    Carrot Colon
        Cleanse, 88–89
    Clean Artery Sweep,
        92–93
    Clean as a Whistle
        Kidney Cleanse,
        90–91
    Garden Fresh Blast,
        94–95
    Great Grapefruit
        Cleanse, 96–97
    Green Joint Relief,
        98–99

Healthy Heart
  Summer Salad,
  112–113
Healthy Prostate
  Blend, 104–105
Heart Beet, 100–101
LDL Reducer, 102–103
Love Boost, 106–107
Under Pressure,
  114–115
Spinach Sugar
  Stabilizer, 108–109
Stimulating
  Sunshine, 110
Get Things Moving,
  144–145
Getting a Boost, 126–127
Ginger, 51
  Achy Breaky
    Muscles, 78
  Acid Away, 136
  Allergy Relief, 200
  Apple Alzheimer's
    Prevention, 224
  Balancing Act, 80
  Beet Cramps, 82
  Beeting Eczema, 240
  Better Body, 162
  Bye-Bye Nausea, 138
  Carrot Colon
    Cleanse, 88
  Citrus Cellulite Be
    Gone, 246
  Clearly Cabbage, 226
  Easy Digestion, 142
  Fat Furnace, 188
  Flu Fighter, 122
  Full System Boost, 124
  Getting a Boost, 126
  Good Morning, 146
  Great Grapefruit
    Cleanse, 96
  Green Heartburn
    Relief, 148
  Green Joint Relief, 98

Happy Colon, 170
Happy in a Glass, 230
Healthful Heart
  Ginger, 172
Healthy Heart
  Summer Salad, 112
Healthy Prostate
  Blend, 104–105
Heart Beet, 100
IBS Support, 152
Inflammation
  Buster, 208
Love Boost, 106
Metabolism Mover,
  156
Minty Fennel, 212
Papaya Gut
  Reprieve, 158
Slow Energy, 196
Splendid Sinuses, 132
Stimulating
  Sunshine, 110
Vanishing Veins, 252
Vital MS Support, 220
Gingerol, 78
Glowing Ginseng,
  206–207
Glycemic index (GI), 196
  ingredients for low
    juices, 197
Good Morning, 146–147
Gout, 168
  ingredients to prevent
    and ease, 169
Gout Be Gone, 168–169
Grapefruit, 26
  Balancing Act, 80
  Citrus Cellulite Be
    Gone, 246
  Citrus Cough
    Buster, 118
  Fat Furnace, 188
  Good Morning, 146
  Great Grapefruit
    Cleanse, 96

Happy Colon, 170
Metabolism Mover,
  156
Grapes, 25, 47
Great Grapefruit Cleanse,
  96–97
Green bell peppers
  Under Pressure, 114
Green Go-Go, 190–191
Green Heartburn Relief,
  148–149
Green Joint Relief, 98–99
Gut flora, 150
  ingredients to build
    good, 151
Gut Flora Builder,
  150–151

**H**

Hair, 248, 250
  ingredients for
    shiny, 251
  ingredients for thick,
    healthy, 249
Halitosis, 54
Happy Colon, 170–171
Happy in a Glass, 230–231
Headaches, 232
  ingredients to prevent
    or ease, 233
Health, ingredients for
  promoting overall
  good, 121
Healthful Headache
  Remedy, 232–233
Healthful Heart Ginger,
  172–173
Healthy Heart Summer
  Salad, 112–113
Healthy Prostate Blend,
  104–105
Heart Beet, 100–101
Heartburn, 148
  ingredients to
    ease, 149

Heart disease, 54, 100, 172, 208
  ingredients to prevent, 173
Heart health, ingredients for, 101
Herbal teas, 16
Herbs and spices, 48–53
High blood pressure, 54, 114
  ingredients to lower, 115
High blood sugar, 108
High cholesterol, 54, 102
Honey
  Sage Advice for Sore Throat, 130
Honeydew, 26
Hormones
  ingredients to help balance, 81
  levels of, 80
Hot peppers, 47
Hydration, 232
  ingredients for, 229
Hydrogen cyanide, 14
Hypothyroidism, 178
  ingredients to prevent and manage, 179

**I**

IBS Support, 152–153
Immune system, 8, 118–133
  Citrus Cough Buster, 118–119
  Flu Fighter, 122–123
  Full System Boost, 124–125
  Getting a Boost, 126–127
  Kick the Cold, 128–129
  Sage Advice for Sore Throat, 130–131
  Splendid Sinuses, 132–133
  Superfood Detox, 120–121
Immunity, ingredients for boosting, 125, 127
Inflammation, 200–221, 208, 214
  Allergy Relief, 200–201
  Asparagus Arthritis Relief, 202–203
  Breathe Easy, 204–205
  Glowing Ginseng, 206–207
  Inflammation Buster, 208–209
  ingredients to prevent and ease, 215
  ingredients to reduce, 209
  Liquid Chlorophyll, 210–211
  Minty Fennel, 212–213
  Passionately Immune, 214–215
  Perky Parsnip, 216–217
  Simply Wheatgrass, 218–219
  Vital MS Support, 220–221
Inflammation Buster, 208–209
Insomnia, 236
  ingredients to prevent, 237
Insulin resistance, 108
Iron, 94
Irritable bowel syndrome (IBS), 152
  ingredients to ease, 153

**J**

Jalapeño pepper
  Beet the Heat, 84
  Better Body, 162
  Garden Fresh Blast, 94
Jicama, 40
  Breathe Easy, 204
Joint pain, ingredients to ease, 99
Juice cleanse, 6, 9, 57–65, 67–74
  amount of juice in, 15
  appropriateness of, 61–62
  benefits of, 59–61
  defined, 57–59
  exercise and, 17, 64
  getting protein with, 15–16
  goal of, 65
  nausea and, 64
  seven-day detox challenge, 71–74
  side effects of, 17
  supplements with, 15
  three-day pure juice cleanse plan, 69–71
  tips for safe and successful, 62–65
Juicer, buying a, 9–12
Juices
  mixing water with, 15
  storage of, 15
  taking premade to work, 16
Juicing
  amount of time doing, 14
  defined, 5–6
  diabetes and, 16
  equipment for, 5
  FAQ about, 13–17
  health benefits of, 6, 7–8, 19

in history, 5
regular, 7
technique tips for,
12–13
tips for, 54–56
weight loss and, 13

# K

Kale, 40, 47
Aftermath Recovery,
182
Carrot Clear-Up, 242
Clean Artery
Sweep, 92
Cutting Cancer, 166
Does a Body Good, 140
Green Go-Go, 190
Green Joint Relief, 98
IBS Support, 152
Love Boost, 106
Papaya Gut
Reprieve, 158
Vital MS Support, 220
Kick the Cold, 128–129
Kidneys, 90
ingredients for
cleansing, 91
Kiwis, 26–27
Bonny Bone Fruit
Surprise, 164
Burn, Baby, Burn, 186
Get Things
Moving, 144
Getting a Boost, 126

# L

LDL cholesterol, 92,
102, 112
LDL Reducer, 102–103
Lemongrass, 41
Lemons, 27
Aftermath Recovery,
182
Allergy Relief, 200
Beeting Eczema, 240

Bladder Infection Be
Gone, 86
Breathe Easy, 204
Bye-Bye Nausea, 138
Carrot Colon
Cleanse, 88
Circle Banisher, 244
Clearly Cabbage, 226
Garden Fresh
Blast, 94
Get Things
Moving, 144
Getting a Boost, 126
Glowing Ginsea, 206
Good Morning, 146
Gout Be Gone, 168
Great Grapefruit
Cleanse, 96
Gut Flora
Builder, 150
Before Gym
Blitz, 184
Healthy Prostate
Blend, 104–105
IBS Support, 152
Inflammation
Buster, 208
Kick the Cold, 128
LDL Reducer, 102
Meal in a Glass, 154
Metabolism Mover,
156
Minty Fennel, 212
Papaya Gut
Reprieve, 158
Rosy Relaxer, 234
Sage Advice for Sore
Throat, 130
Shiny Tresses, 250
Simply Wheatgrass,
218
Slow Energy, 196
Splendid Sinuses, 132
Stimulating
Sunshine, 110

Superfood Detox, 120
Sweet Dreams, 236
Thyroid Buddy, 178
Vanishing Veins, 252
Lettuce, 41, 47. *See also*
Romaine lettuce
Leukemia, 162
ingredients to
fight, 163
Libido, 8, 106
ingredients for
increased, 107
Limes, 27
Apple Alzheimer's
Prevention, 224
Better Body, 162
Citrus Cellulite Be
Gone, 246
Citrus Cough
Buster, 118
Clean Artery
Sweep, 92
Clean as a Whistle
Kidney Cleanse, 90
Green Go-Go, 190
Happy Colon, 170
Healthy Prostate
Blend, 104–105
Promote Prostate
Health, 174
Stimulating
Sunshine, 110
Liquid Chlorophyll,
210–211
Liver, 84, 96
ingredients to cleanse
the, 85, 97
Lots of Locks, 248–249
Love Boost, 106–107
Lutein, 112
Lycopene, 104, 110, 174

# M

Magnesium, 172, 230
Maintenance diet, 140

Male sexual function,
ingredients to
support, 111
Malic acid, 142
Mangoes, 27
Masticating juicers, 11
Meal in a Glass, 154–155
Memory, 8
Menstrual cramps, 82
ingredients to
prevent or ease, 83
Mental clarity, 226
ingredients for, 227
Mental fog, 228
Metabolic syndrome, 108
Metabolism, 156, 186
ingredients for
boosting, 157, 187
Metabolism Mover,
156–157
Mind, brain, and mental
wellness, 224–237
Apple Alzheimer's
Prevention,
224–225
Clearly Cabbage,
226–227
Focus on Hydration,
228–229
Happy in a Glass,
230–231
Healthful Headache
Remedy, 232–233
Rosy Relaxer, 234–235
Sweet Dreams,
236–237
Mint, 51
Achy Breaky
Muscles, 78
Beet Cramps, 82
Bonny Bone Fruit
Surprise, 164
Focus on
Hydration, 228
Before Gym Blitz, 184

Minty Fennel, 212
Minty Fennel, 212–213
Mood, ingredients to
boost, 231
Morning sickness, 146
ingredients to
ease, 147
Multiple sclerosis, 220
ingredients to cope
with, 221
Muscles
ingredients for
recovery of, 195
ingredients to ease
aching, 79
Mustard seed, 51–52

**N**

Nausea, 138
ingredients to
relieve, 139
juice cleanse and, 64
Nectarines, 28, 47
Nutmeg
Inflammation
Buster, 208
Sweet Dreams, 236

**O**

Oleocanthal, 202
Olive oil, 202
Onions, 41–42
Lots of Locks, 248
Orange bell peppers
Cutting Cancer, 166
Oranges, 28
Achy Breaky
Muscles, 78
Citrus Cellulite Be
Gone, 246
Citrus Cough
Buster, 118
Does a Body Good, 140
Fat Furnace, 188
Happy Colon, 170

Passionately
Immune, 214
Ready to Recover, 194
Sage Advice for Sore
Throat, 130
Shiny Tresses, 250
Splendid Sinuses, 132
Organic produce, buying, 16
Osteoporosis, 164
ingredients to
prevent, 165
Oxidation, 8

**P**

Papayas, 28-29
Focus on
Hydration, 228
Healthful Heart
Ginger, 172
Papaya Gut
Reprieve, 158
Papaya Gut Reprieve,
158–159
Parsley, 52
Acid Away, 136
Allergy Relief, 200
Asparagus Arthritis
Relief, 202
Beet Cramps, 82
Beeting Eczema, 240
Breathe Easy, 204
Circle Banisher, 244
Clean as a Whistle
Kidney Cleanse, 90
Full System Boost, 124
Garden Fresh
Blast, 94
Green Go-Go, 190
Green Joint Relief, 98
Healthful Heart
Ginger, 172
Healthy Heart
Summer Salad, 112
Healthy Prostate
Blend, 104–105

IBS Support, 152
Liquid Chlorophyll, 210
Perky Parsnip, 216
Under Pressure, 114
Rosy Relaxer, 234
Slow Energy, 196
Spinach Sugar Stabilizer, 108
Superfood Detox, 120
Sweet Dreams, 236
Parsnips, 42
Kick the Cold, 128
Perky Parsnip, 216
Passionately Immune, 214–215
Passion fruit, 29
Passionately Immune, 214
Peaches, 29, 47
Pears, 29–30, 47
Bonny Bone Fruit Surprise, 164
Bye-Bye Nausea, 138
Green Go-Go, 190
Green Joint Relief, 98
Happy in a Glass, 230
Healthful Headache Remedy, 232
Healthful Heart Ginger, 172
Heart Beet, 100
Inflammation Buster, 208
Meal in a Glass, 154
Perky Parsnip, 216
Peas, 42
Pectin, 140
Peppers. See Cayenne pepper; Green bell peppers; Jalapeño pepper; Orange bell peppers; Red bell peppers
Perky Parsnip, 216–217

Pesticides, 45–47
testing of fruits and vegetables for, 46–47
Phytonutrients, 100
Pick Me Up, 192–193
Pineapple, 30
Allergy Relief, 200
Bonny Bone Fruit Surprise, 164
Burn, Baby, Burn, 186
Inflammation Buster, 208
Sage Advice for Sore Throat, 130
Vanishing Veins, 252
Plums, 30, 47
Polyphenol, 102, 192
Post-workout recovery, ingredients for better, 183
Potassium, 114, 172
Potatoes, 47
Prebiotics, 150
Progesterone, 80
Promote Prostate Health, 174–175
Prostate cancer, 104, 174
ingredients to prevent, 175
Prostate health, 104
ingredients for, 105
Protein, getting, with juice cleanse, 15–16
Pumpkin, 31
Glowing Ginseng, 206
Pick Me Up, 192

Q
Quercetin, 204, 224

R
Radishes, 43
Fat Furnace, 188
Kick the Cold, 128

Raspberries, 31
Ready to Recover, 194–195
Red bell peppers
Breathe Easy, 204
Garden Fresh Blast, 94
Glowing Ginseng, 206
Kick the Cold, 128
Rosy Relaxer, 234
Regularity, ingredients to promote, 145
Rheumatoid arthritis, 216
ingredients to prevent and ease, 217
Romaine lettuce
Achy Breaky Muscles, 78
Before Gym Blitz, 184
Rosemary, 52
Rosy Relaxer, 234–235

S
Sage, 52–53, 130
Sage Advice for Sore Throat, 130
Sage Advice for Sore Throat, 130–131
Selenium, 204
Seven-day detox challenge, 71–74
Sexual health, 110
Shiny Tresses, 250–251
Simply Wheatgrass, 218–219
Single-gear juicers, 11
Sinus allergies, 200
Sinusitis, ingredients for, 133
Slow Energy, 196–197
Snap peas, 47
Sore throat, ingredients to fight, 131
Spinach, 10, 43–44, 47
Acid Away, 136
Aftermath Recovery, 182

Beet Cramps, 82
Beet the Heat, 84
Better Body, 162
Bye-Bye Nausea, 138
Circle Banisher, 244
Citrus Cough
    Buster, 118
Clearly Cabbage, 226
Flu Fighter, 122
Garden Fresh
    Blast, 94
Get Things
    Moving, 144
Getting a Boost, 126
Green Go-Go, 190
Before Gym Blitz, 184
Healthful Heart
    Ginger, 172
Healthy Heart
    Summer Salad, 112
Healthy Prostate
    Blend, 104–105
Lots of Locks, 248
Pick Me Up, 192
Spinach Sugar
    Stabilizer, 108
Under Pressure, 114
Stimulating Sunshine, 110
Spinach Sugar Stabilizer,
    108–109
Splendid Sinuses, 132–133
Squash. See
    Butternut squash
Stimulating Sunshine, 110
Strawberries, 31–32, 47
    Shiny Tresses, 250
Superfood Detox, 120–121
Supplements with juice
    cleanse, 15
Sweet bell peppers, 47
Sweet Dreams, 236–237
Sweet potatoes, 43
    Breathe Easy, 204
    Passionately
        Immune, 214

Shiny Tresses, 250
Swiss chard, 44
    Full System Boost, 124
    LDL Reducer, 102
    Shiny Tresses, 250

T

Tangerines, 32
Three-day pure juice
    cleanse plan, 69–71
Thyme, 53
    Apple Alzheimer's
        Prevention, 224
    Circle Banisher, 244
    Perky Parsnip, 216
Thyroid, 178
Thyroid Buddy, 178–179
Tomatoes, 32
    Garden Fresh Blast, 94
    Healthy Prostate
        Blend, 104–105
    Meal in a Glass, 154
    Under Pressure, 114
    Rosy Relaxer, 234
    Stimulating
        Sunshine, 110
Toxins, 45–47
Triturating juicers, 11–12
Turmeric, 53
    Great Grapefruit
        Cleanse, 96
    Liquid Chlorophyll,
        210
    Stimulating
        Sunshine, 110
Turnips, 44

U

Ulcerative colitis, 212
    ingredients to ease
        and prevent, 213
Under Pressure, 114–115
Uric acid, 168
Urinary tract
    infections, 86

ingredients to
    prevent or treat, 87
Urine, color of, 16

V

Vanishing Veins, 252–253
Varicose veins, 252
    ingredients to
        prevent, 253
Vegetable juice, versus
    fruit juice, 20–21
Vegetables, 13, 33–45. See
    also specific
Vital MS Support, 220–221
Vitamin A, 118
Vitamin C, 8, 118, 126, 130,
    164, 172
Vitamin D, 164
Vitamin E, 8, 126

W

Water, mixing with
    juices, 15
Watercress
    Sweet Dreams, 236
    Thyroid Buddy, 178
Watermelon, 33
    Achy Breaky
        Muscles, 78
    Clean as a Whistle
        Kidney Cleanse, 90
    Focus on
        Hydration, 228
    Promote Prostate
        Health, 174
Weight loss, 13, 154
    ingredients to
        promote, 155
Weight loss and digestion
    enhancers, 136–159
    Acid Away, 136–137
    Bye-Bye Nausea,
        138–139
    Does a Body Good,
        140–141

Easy Digestion,
142–143
Get Things Moving,
144–145
Good Morning,
146–147
Green Heartburn
Relief, 148–149
Gut Flora Builder,
150–151
IBS Support,
152–153
Meal in a Glass,
154–155

Metabolism Mover,
156–157
Papaya Gut Reprieve,
158–159
Weight maintenance, 140
ingredients for, 141
Wheatgrass, 45
Liquid Chlorophyll,
210
Simply Wheatgrass,
218
Workout
ingredients for before
a, 185

ingredients for post
recovery, 183
ingredients for
stamina, 191

**Y**

Yellow bell peppers
Burn, Baby, Burn, 186
Vanishing Veins, 252

**Z**

Zucchini, 45
Does a Body Good,
140